Lose Your Menopause Belly

The Simple 4 Step System to Lose the Fat and Get Your Sexy Back After 40

Author:

Shawna Kaminski BEd, BKin, MTT

Foreword

The Power of Persistence and Positive People

By Craig Ballantyne

Author, The Perfect Day Formula

You know the old joke.

"How do you eat an elephant?"

The answer.

"One bite at a time."

It doesn't matter what your circumstances in life. You might be struggling with hormonal issues, family squabbles, office drama, or a little extra belly fat hanging on to your bikini belly.

All of these problems can be overcome with persistent and positive people.

I know because one of my friends is living proof.

Her name is Shawna Kaminski, and today she's a powerful inspiration to millions of women around the world.

But when I first met her, Shawna was as timid as a church mouse. Sure, her intelligence, empathy, and expertise were as clear as day, but she held herself back from having a massive impact.

Fortunately, she just needed a little confidence and experience.

Even better, Shawna doesn't know the meaning of the word, "quit." She conquered unruly students over her two-decade career as a teacher. She raised two children into fine, upstanding adults who will have a big impact of their own someday. She weathered the storm of a broken marriage, as so many of us must do. And throughout all of this, no matter how busy she was, she made time for her health and fitness and what really mattered in her life.

Those are just a few of the reasons you've wisely chosen her to be the role model for your life.

Shawna's life isn't easy today. She juggles her multiple

fitness businesses and fitness bootcamp location. She continues her personal and professional growth in many areas. And she's constantly vigilant of her children, making sure they stay on track as they leave the nest.

Her persistence is a key to her success, but so are the people she surrounds herself with in her personal and professional life.

Full disclosure, Shawna is a coaching client of mine. I've been her business mentor for going on eight years. (Wow, eight years... where has the time gone!?!)

As a coach, I bring Shawna two things that no one else can provide. First, there is expert advice. Just as you go to Shawna, a world-class expert in helping women over 40 lose weight and get back in shape, Shawna looks to me for advice in helping her publish books, create videos, and positively impact millions of lives every year.

Second, and perhaps more importantly, I give Shawna no-excuse accountability. I hold her to higher standards than anyone else expects from her. I see what she is capable of achieving, and if she doesn't live up to those expectations, we have a heart-to-heart discussion about what needs to change.

All of this is done in her best interests.

This is how she turned from timid church mouse into

world-renowned leader and motivational force to women in over 100 countries around the globe.

That's the power of persistence and positive people.

And these pillars will work for you, too.

If you're looking for fast, incredible results in every area of your life, then your best decision would be to get expert advice, accountability, and support from Shawna.

There's no one better in the world, no one more qualified, no one more capable, and no one more caring than Shawna Kaminski.

She'll be the most positive person in your life. She'll make sure you persist through the tough times. She'll help you finally achieve your big goals and dreams – the ones that you desire and deserve.

Your time is now. Your leader is here.

Follow Shawna.

She'll change your life.

Just like she changed hers.

To your success.

Table of Contents

Chapter 1 - HELP Is On the Way! 1

Chapter 2 – Menopause Myth Busting 19

Chapter 3 - How Does Exercise Help? 37

Chapter 4 – Make Your Nutrition Count 55

Chapter 5 – Sleep and Other Menopause Mysteries ... 89

Chapter 6 – Mindset Magic 99

Chapter 7 – Work with Me 117

Chapter 1 - HELP Is On the Way!

If you can change the way people think, the way they see themselves, the way they see the world, if you can do that, you can change the way people live their lives. That's the only lasting thing you can create.

Chuck Palahniuk

Warning: If you believe that suffering through menopause symptoms is a fact of life, YOU ARE WRONG. You are needlessly suffering and even putting your health at risk.

Can you say YES to two or more of these frustrations?

- You have little time to take care of yourself and your expanding waistline...

- You can't fall asleep, stay asleep and you wake up burning hot.

- You can no longer lose 5 lbs as quickly as you did

when you were 30 and the weight just seems to be piling up around your belly.

- You starve yourself and you even gain weight eating nothing but salads.

- You're plagued with injury, aches and pains.

- You're frustrated with long workouts, expensive gym memberships and personal trainers.

- You feel burdened with responsibility as you're sandwiched between caring for your growing children and aging parents.

- Every day you feel like you're losing control and things will never get better.

- You wonder what happened to the 'old you'…

It's likely that you and the majority of women would blame most of these woes on menopause, but guess what? It's likely that something entirely different than menopause is your issue.

Yes, that's right.

Menopause is taking the blame, but it's actually something called ***somatopause*** that's contributing to your menopausal symptoms and keeping you from living the life you desire.

Somatopause is REAL.

More on somatopause in a moment, but first, an introduction is in order…

I'm Shawna K and I know exactly what you're going through…I'm living in your shoes. I'm in my early 50's and I totally understand your frustrations.

But I've helped thousands of women just like you discover the solution.

So today, there's great news for you, but first the bad news…

The fact is, if you continue on this path, your energy, confidence and ability to live the life you want in the healthy body you desire declines a little more each day.

In fact, this decline can hit once you reach the age of 30 years old.

This downward spiral is called *'somatopause'* and it all starts when an important anti-aging hormone called HGH (or Human Growth Hormone) levels begin to drop dramatically.

Why is this a big deal?

This decline of HGH is part of what drives the aging process. Somatopause and all these frustrations are NOT your fault.

You've been fed MISINFORMATION regarding menopause and healthy aging.

After all, have you even heard about somatopause before? Probably not.

You don't have to accept a menopause belly, a tanking metabolism, low energy, mood swings and every other 'symptom' fed to us by the media and millennials that simply write us off as 'old' and worn out.

> STUDIES HAVE SHOWN THAT ASIAN WOMEN TRADITIONALLY HAVE NOT EXPERIENCED MANY OF THE MENOPAUSAL SYMPTOMS THAT WE ARE TOLD ARE INEVITABLE. IN FACT, THE JAPANESE DON'T EVEN HAVE A WORD FOR HOT FLASHES! IT'S ONLY BEEN IN RECENT YEARS SINCE ASIAN WOMEN HAVE ADOPTED WESTERN FOOD AND LIFESTYLES THAT THEY TOO ARE STARTING TO EXPERIENCE SIMILAR MENOPAUSAL FRUSTRATIONS.

References: Melby MK. Vasomotor symptom prevalence and language of menopause in Japan. Menopause. 2005;12(3):250-257. Chim H, Tan BH, Ang CC, Chew EM, Chong YS, Saw SM. The prevalence of menopausal symptoms in a community in Singapore. Maturitas. 2002;41(4):275-282.

The GOOD NEWS is that you can take control of your health with less effort than you think. There's a 'gene therapy' also known as epigenetics, that you can employ so you can be as healthy and vibrant as you've ever been.

You can actually start to reverse the signs of aging so that you can enjoy the things you love. You can rid yourself of that unwanted midlife belly bulge and experience steady, sustainable fat loss and stop 'dieting' forever.

In fact, ANY woman at ANY age can discover how to get a flat and firm attractive stomach - Even If NOTHING has worked in the past. And you can increase your confidence and energy so you'll be the person you want to be, not just a shell of a person going through the motions of life.

The concepts in this book will help you to permanently banish belly fat and put a serious dent in your frustrating menopausal symptoms.

Sometimes people ask: Would you turn back the clock if you could? My answer is 'No way!'.

Even though we have a faster metabolism in our 20's, you and I would never trade our life experience and wisdom.

You're about to discover my secrets to feel the very best in your own skin.

When you do, you'll experience the 'ripple effect'.

An empowered and healthy woman affects her partner, her children, her co-workers and friends. In fact, this secret will not only help you, it will help 6-8 more people in your circle through this ripple effect. Women like YOU will change the world to make it a healthier and more positive place.

Take Claudia for example, this is what she has to say about using my secrets:

> Once I started exercising with Shawna, my family saw how energized and healthy I became and wanted to join in too. Now we love to exercise together as a family.

> *Claudia O.*

And I want to share my secrets with you.

After all, *somatopause is the enemy NOT menopause.*

You may think that we need to find a CURE for menopause, but menopause is just a natural part of aging that isn't necessarily the culprit to our woes.

In fact, we can't 'cure' menopause anymore than we can 'cure' puberty.

However, I have some solutions to somatopause, which will ease our menopausal symptoms.

And gene therapy is the answer….

Let me tell you a little about how this gene therapy

breakthrough, called *epigenetics*, will help ease our way through the natural shift in hormones known as menopause.

But first, I want to share a compelling story with you from one of my clients, I'll call her 'Rachel' – it's very personal and it was a challenge for her to put down on paper. I encouraged her to allow me to share it here with you because I KNOW you'll resonate with it.

I want you to see how she turned her life around by harnessing the power of gene therapy to defeat somatopause, lose her belly fat and ease her menopausal symptoms.

When Rachel turned 40, her world started to crash down….

She looked around and believed everyone was thinner, prettier, happier, more successful, and BETTER than her. She sank into a spiral of depression, sickness and weight gain…

Rachel was successful in all other aspects of her life.

She started drinking more wine than she would like to admit and ate too much chocolate.

Her exercise dwindled to barely anything.

Outwardly things looked 'normal', however her hormones were all over the place. She was experiencing wild mood swings, anger and an ever-expanding waistline.

Her husband was growing distant and she was so afraid he'd leave her.

And her weight kept climbing.

She was tired and sluggish all the time. Every physical activity, even her favorite past-time of gardening was a huge effort.

She was ashamed.

She felt shame that she was out of control with her eating and drinking. She was hooked on anything that gave her an immediate sugar high and she didn't worry about the inevitable crash that came later.

She felt like a drug addict, except that her drug of choice was food.

She felt invisible, even though she had put on 60 pounds in less than 2 years.

Her skin was dull and blotchy and none of her clothes fit. She was a mess.....

Does any part of this story sound familiar?

Let me tell you about how gene therapy (or epigenetics) helped Rachel turn her life around and how epigenetics can help YOU combat somatopause too.

Somatopause can be stopped in its tracks when we implement scientifically engineered exercise sequences. Period.

> NEW RESEARCH PUBLISHED IN THE JOURNAL CELL METABOLISM SHOWS THAT EVEN BRIEF EXERCISE PRODUCES AN IMMEDIATE CHANGE IN DNA. EXERCISE CAUSES IMPORTANT STRUCTURAL AND CHEMICAL CHANGES TO THE DNA MOLECULES WITHIN MUSCLES.
>
> THIS STUDY SUGGESTS THAT WHEN WE EXERCISE, OUR BODY ALMOST IMMEDIATELY EXPERIENCES GENETIC ACTIVATION THAT INCREASES THE PRODUCTION OF FAT-BUSTING PROTEINS.

We will experience greater fat loss results in less time and with less effort when we implement these specific scientifically engineered exercise sequences.

We can forget about our bad genetics because this gene therapy or EPIGENETIC modification can actually help us change our cells from the inside out.

The result of this exercise will be an elevation of your natural HGH (human growth hormone) levels. And remember, declining HGH levels are the root of all age related issues.

MENOPAUSE SYMPTOMS SUCH AS HOT FLASHES, NIGHT SWEATS, IRRITABILITY, BRAIN FOG AND OTHER SYMPTOMS SEEM TO BE CONSIDERED THE NORM FOR WOMEN OVER THE AGE OF 50.

RESEARCHERS FROM THE DEPARTMENT OF INTEGRATED HEALTH AT WESTMINSTER UNIVERSITY POLLED 1,000 BRITISH WOMEN AGES 45 TO 55 AND COMPARED THEIR ANSWERS TO THOSE OF WOMEN FROM THE U.S., CANADA, JAPAN AND CHINA.

THE CONCLUSION WAS THAT JAPANESE AND CHINESE WOMEN SUFFER THE LEAST AMOUNT OF MENOPAUSE SYMPTOMS. THE REASONS FOR THESE CULTURAL DIFFERENCES ARE COMPLEX. CERTAINLY DIET AND LIFESTYLE CHOICES PLAY A KEY ROLE.

BRITISH WOMEN SUFFER THE MOST AND NORTH AMERICANS ARE SOMEWHERE IN BETWEEN.

WHILE THE EXACT REASONS FOR INCREASED MENOPAUSAL SYMPTOMS AREN'T ENTIRELY CLEAR, MAYBE IT'S AS SIMPLE AS ASIAN WOMEN UNDERSTANDING ""LET FOOD BE THY MEDICINE AND MEDICINE BE THY FOOD."

BOTTOM LINE? DIET AND EXERCISE PLAY AN INCREASINGLY IMPORTANT ROLE IN RELIEF OF MENOPAUSAL SYMPTOMS IN WOMEN OVER 40.

That's what Rachel experienced; I'll let her explain it:

I was helplessly out of control and I couldn't see a way to get myself back on track until one day I asked for help.

I found a coach who specialized in women's health and fitness over the age of 35. And she showed me in simple steps how to reclaim control of my eating and she showed me how to begin to exercise.

With each simple success, no matter how small, my confidence started to grow.

At first the exercise bouts seemed difficult because they were foreign and new, but each short workout got easier so that I actually looked forward to them.

I was thrilled to see:

- My hormones finally started to stabilize.
- My body started to change.
- My mind started to change.
- I started to feel pride in my efforts.

And as I progressed, slowly the weight crept off.

I knew I had to stop comparing my progress with others. I had to let go of past weight loss failures, having tried everything under the sun. I knew I had to stay the course.

I wanted to stop dieting and start living.

Life became easier as I embraced my newfound healthy habits.

Within five months of moving more and eating cleaner, I was able to get off the medication I'd relied on for five years.

My skin cleared, my migraines had almost stopped, I lost 17 pounds of body fat and I dropped 2 dress sizes.

Another happy result was that as I developed a whole host of healthy habits, my entire family adopted them too!

Thank you to my mentor and coach, Shawna K for giving me my life back.

Science proves that EXERCISE is the real FOUNTAIN OF YOUTH boosting our body's natural production of human growth hormone (HGH).

Exercise addresses SOMATOPAUSE - the root cause of serious muscle loss and atrophy that typically occurs with aging. When you address our decreasing HGH levels, we'll look and feel younger for longer and stay healthier and stronger while we even FIX OUR MENOPAUSE BELLY.

Exercise will literally change us from the inside out.

A 2011 REVIEW IN APPLIED PHYSIOLOGY, NUTRITION AND METABOLISM POINTS OUT THAT EXERCISE INCREASES YOUR METABOLISM SO WE'LL BURN MORE CALORIES DOING LESS ACTIVITY.

Feeling sluggish? The studies show that benefits are far reaching: specific exercise sequences not only make us leaner but we'll also feel more energized.

Are you forgetful? At least two additional studies, one in the Journal of Applied Physiology and the other in Neuroscience, also showed that exercise can even change the brain so that potential benefits such as reduction or reversal of age-associated declines in cognitive function can occur.

There's more than enough compelling evidence to show that the right exercise is THE ANSWER to combating the REAL enemy of somatopause. And by doing so, menopausal symptoms are relieved.

Rachel used MY scientifically engineered exercise sequences and literally fixed her menopause belly and that changed her life.

Ever heard of the saying 'how you do anything is how you do everything?' Well, Rachel's menopause belly and her lack of confidence in her body led to her eating binges, her weight gain, her depression, her lethargy.

It was a vicious cycle.

The cycle needed to STOP and she was able to do it with my secrets that balanced her hormones to banish somatopause for good.

An amazing transformation occurs when we commit to ONLY 15-20 minutes of exercise every second day.

Here are the benefits of this small time and energy investment:

- HGH levels are boosted to slow down the aging process.
- Insulin levels are stabilized so you aren't famished or on a rollercoaster of energy surges and crashes.
- The 'happy hormones' (serotonin and dopamine) levels are naturally increased so your mood is uplifted.
- Weight loss occurs slowly and steadily.

If you're interested in sailing through menopause without the weight gain, lethargy, mood swings, sleep disruptions, night sweats and everything else associated with it, , then you're in the right place…

YOU can experience results just like these women:

"I lost 10kg doing this program"

"As an 'older woman' I realize the importance of keeping fit and with this program I know that I can maintain my fitness levels into the future for years to come. I also lost 10kg doing this program by following the nutrition guidelines, by removing the processed 'junk', improving the quality of my food and still enjoying a glass of red wine nightly. I highly recommend this program to anyone who wants to improve their fitness and maintain good health and have fun at the same time!"

Elizabeth Phillips, 68

"The workouts were really motivational"

"I improved my strength, fitness and joint mobility. The workouts were really motivational and taught me correct technique to prevent injury. I have to be very careful of my wrists and these exercises allowed me to do that but still have a challenging workout."

Lynda Smith, 63

Whether you have 10, 20, 30 or more pounds to lose, this book will guide and support you the entire way.

Put the PAUSE on MENOPAUSE for good.

I'm not suggesting a complicated exercise plan that will leave you exhausted while tearing apart your joints with dangerous high impact exercises….

And I'm not suggesting that you have to "starve yourself skinny" on some outrageous diet that makes you miserable only to gain ALL the weight back and more once you go back to eating normally…

But we can use epigenetics to put the brakes on somatopause.

If you're menopausal, your symptoms will be eased as you start to change your body from the inside out. You'll balance your hormones to get off the hormonal rollercoaster.

Or if you're not close to menopause, you'll balance your hormones and acquire a more favourable body composition NOW so that menopause symptoms are hardly an issue.

You can experience steady, sustainable fat loss so that you can stop 'dieting' and start living. And you can flatten and firm your belly while REVERSING dangerous diseases like heart hypertension, cardiovascular disease, and even diabetes without any pills or expensive medications…

Are you excited yet? You should be!

In the next chapter, I'll dig into some menopause myths so you'll really understand from a physiological point of view what's going on inside your body that's causing your menopause belly.

But don't worry, it's an easy read – no medical training required.

After that, we'll dig into the 4 simple steps to lose your menopause belly:

1. Adding the 'right' exercise

2. Eating the 'right' foods

3. Sleeping 'right'

4. Thinking the 'right' thoughts

Let's get started!

Chapter 2 – Menopause Myth Busting

It's amazing what a woman on fire can accomplish!

Sharon Hodor Greenthal

It's fair to argue now that we can straight up stop blaming our menopause belly on menopause alone. It turns out that other factors, one of which is somatopause, is likely MORE to blame.

But either way, no matter what or who the culprit is, you might have this belly and you want to get rid of it, right?

I want to encourage you. I want to remind you that it's entirely possible to change your body, well into our 40's, 50's and beyond.

Let me share Suzie Salmon's story with you. It's a '25 pound weight loss journey'....

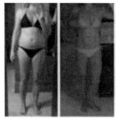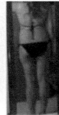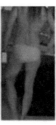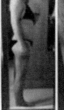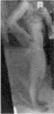

Prior to working with me and my style of workouts, Suzie had gained 25 pounds in a year. She came to this realization:

"I have to say the toughest part of changing my ways was actually leading myself out of denial and making up MY MIND that it was time to do something"

Initially she started to run to meet her goals. She ran because she LOVED running but she was disappointed with the results. Running just didn't cut it the way it once did to get the body she had hoped for. Not only this, her running brought on an insatiable hunger and NO weight came off (she actually gained weight).

She realized that she was interested in MORE than just weight loss. Her goals changed to these:

- She wanted **health**, **life** and **strength**.
- She realized her mental health was just as important as her physical health.

- She found the roadblock, set her goals, and clarified her intentions so that she started to hold herself accountable.

And that's when the magic really happened.

She started to do my style of workouts up to six days a week. Workouts were only 15-20 minutes in length and used her bodyweight as resistance and a whole lot of science to deliver a kick butt metabolically challenging workout at home. Some days the workout were as short as 8-10 minutes.

She said, 'There's so much variety to my workouts that I'm never bored! Trust me, I get bored REALLY fast! So I think this is why I am still sticking to the program. My long workouts are 30-45 minutes, depending on whether I add a 4-6 minute **'body sculpt workout'** onto the end, and every other day they're short. I get in, get out, and get 'er done! **And in 20 weeks, I haven't missed a workout…**now that's consistency!'

Did she change how she ate?

Suzie is a nutritional anthropologist so she understands nutrition as it relates to health. What she loves about how she eats now is that it's delicious, nutritious, filling and it's REAL food. She eats 'clean' 80-90% of the time and lives her life 100% of the time as a result of it. She eats for performance, that is, she wanted to feel energized and strong. Luckily, losing weight and inches was a happy coincidence.

So what has Suzie's progress been so far?

In 20 weeks of following the program, Suzie has managed to trim over 20 inches and she's also lost 25.4 lb.

More importantly, Suzie gained muscle, tone and control of her life.

So…here's what she likes the most about this change:

- She doesn't consider her nutritional changes a 'diet'.

- Suzie has made a lifestyle change and one that fits HER lifestyle. She's able to get her workouts done in under 30 minutes when SHE wants to at home.

- She makes healthy choices for eating and training a priority.

I'm super proud of Suzie and the progress she's made. An added benefit is that many people in Suzie's life have followed her lead to become more fit.

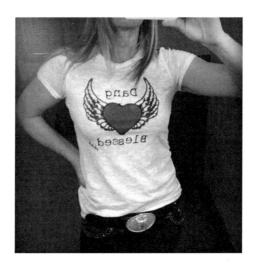

Suzie is feeling good in her jeans again (and looking fantastic if you ask me)

Suzie's results aren't unusual. You can get similar results when you implement my strategies.

Now, let's get started with busting some menopause myths. I'll address some of the common questions and comments I get asked.

'I turned 40 and my metabolism tanked. It must be the start of menopause!'

Many people mistakenly think, "I'm turning 40 or once

I start perimenopause my metabolism is just going to tank."

So, does metabolism really slow down at menopause?

This isn't necessarily the case – *and that's good news* – keep reading and you'll find out why.

The change in metabolism actually happens even before perimenopause approaches. This metabolic slowdown isn't really related to your menopause hormones at all. In fact, *lifestyle* has more to do with midlife weight gain than menopause.

Interestingly enough, take a look around and you'll see that many men are experiencing some of the same belly fat weight gain as women.

So, it's not just women that gain belly fat as we age. Menopause hormones play only a minor role to weight gain. Remember what I said about somatopause? Men suffer from it too.

What's causing this metabolic slowdown in the 40's?

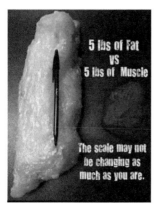

As I just mentioned, it's more your lifestyle and the loss of lean muscle that causes a metabolic tanking than actually menopause.

This is a surprise to a lot of people. Take a look at this image:

This image displays five pounds of fat and five pounds of muscle.

Now I always laugh when people say, "Well, muscle weighs more than fat" because these both weigh five pounds.

What people actually mean is that the *density* of muscle and fat is different.

Muscle will take up less space in your jeans if you have five pounds of fat compared to five pounds of muscle on your frame. You're going to slip into your jeans much easier when you have a little more muscle on your body.

The scale doesn't always tell the whole story.

We shouldn't just judge by what the scale says because it's actually *body composition* that makes a big difference in how we look and feel.

Typically, most people's composition changes in our 30's. This sets us up to think that by the 40's, the metabolism is slowing down and menopause is hitting.

It's actually not that menopause is hitting so much, it's more that we've lost some of our lean muscle. This is because often we become more sedentary, and as we become more sedentary we lose muscle tone. This has everything to do with somatopause and not much to do with menopause.

Even if our body weight stays the same, our body composition has more than likely changed.

For example, let's say you are 150 pounds at age 30. If you're lucky to maintain that same weight at age 40, you might not be the same composition. The majority of people will have less muscle and more fat – your shape has changed over time. Sadly, it might be akin to a melting candle.

Muscle is shapely and more metabolically active.

Muscle burns more calories even at rest.

Muscle puts the sexy in our jeans.

Sadly, fat is actually just 'dead weight' that requires fewer calories to maintain. As people age, with a sedentary lifestyle, we tend to trade in our lean muscle tone for the 'dead weight' of body fat.

It's typical that as most approach the age of 40, they have gained a little weight – but it's not likely that they've gained more muscle tone, but rather, they've added unsightly fat.

Even if you gain only two pounds a year, which isn't much at all, that's a 20-pound weight gain in 10 years.

This is a double whammy of metabolic slowdown: you have more (less metabolically active) fat on your body and you have less (calorie burning and metabolically active) muscle that has the potential to burn off fat.

The result is you are fatter, softer and you usually don't like the image reflected in the mirror.

Has this happened to you?

Do you weigh a little more now?

Would you be able to say that you have more muscle on your body now than what you did at age 30? Sadly, most would have to agree that you have a little more flub now than 10 years ago.

So, now we've established that weight gain can be a result of lifestyle and not just menopause, I hope you agree that this is FANTASTIC news! It puts you in the driver seat to make necessary changes to reverse this process.

Menopause does have some effect on your metabolism, but it's not the ONLY reason for weight gain. Somatopause, or the reduction of the youth hormone HGH, along with the loss of lean muscle is probably more to blame.

Let's not blame menopause for everything!

It's never too late to make a few simple lifestyle changes. In fact, menopausal symptoms can be reduced with very small consistent efforts over time. Keep reading and I'll go over ways to safely and effectively lose the extra flub around your middle.

What's going on with our hormones?

I often get asked, 'What's going on at menopause that causes abdominal weight gain?'

In this case, we can point the finger at our declining menopause hormones to a certain extent.

The 'minor' issue is that with age, our ovaries produce less estrogen. Fat cells generate estrogen so the body tries harder to convert calories into fat to generate more estrogen. Since the body prefers 'homeostasis' or keeping things the same - as our estrogen levels naturally decreases with age, our body tries to keep estrogen levels 'the same' by producing belly fat filled with estrogen. The more visceral fat, or fat around our belly and organs, the more estrogen your body produces.

This is not a major player in the increase of belly fat. If we can keep other issues in check, we can minimize the effect of this hormonal decline that causes belly fat storage.

Why do we gain weight around the middle?

Many women are battling the inner tire. The common complaint that I hear is:

'My waist is increasing.'

'My jeans don't fit.'

'I used to gain fat on my booty but now it's on my belly and back.'

'I have a muffin top.'

As we age and our estrogen production declines, we have more visceral fat. Visceral fat is the fat that's located around the organs, around our abdomen and inside the abdominal cavity.

Visceral fat is the 'dangerous fat' associated with heart

disease. Obviously we want to be able to keep our visceral fat lower for both aesthetic and health related reasons.

Visceral fat is also associated with following a low fat, high carbohydrate diet and is also associated with insulin resistance. I'll be discussing insulin resistance in another chapter.

In addition, we also may have elevated stress levels that contribute to belly fat accumulation.

What's stress got to do with it?

Our lives are busy and stressful. We are often sandwiched between caring for children, teenagers and/or young adults as well as aging parents. When is there a moment for us?

When we experience high stress levels, our body reacts by flooding itself with cortisol. Our bodies are created for survival and how it reacts to stress is a beautiful illustration.

Our body is hardwired to react to stress in ways meant to protect us against threats from predators and other aggressors. It's unlikely that we face such threats today, but our body reacts similarly.

In fact, our body treats even minor hassles and stresses

as threats. As a result we may feel as if we're constantly under assault.

When we encounter a perceived threat — a large dog barks at us during our morning walk, for instance — our hypothalamus, a tiny region at the base of our brain, sets off an alarm system in our body. Through a combination of nerve and hormonal signals, this system prompts the adrenal glands, located atop our kidneys, to release a surge of hormones, including adrenaline and cortisol.

Adrenaline increases your heart rate, elevates blood pressure and boosts energy supplies. Cortisol, the primary stress hormone, increases sugars (glucose) in the bloodstream, enhances the brain's use of glucose and increases the availability of substances that repair tissues. Our body is getting ready to 'run' or 'fight'.

Cortisol also curbs functions that would be nonessential or detrimental in a fight-or-flight situation. It alters immune system responses and suppresses the digestive system, the reproductive system and growth processes. This complex natural alarm system also communicates with regions of our brain that control mood, motivation and fear.

The body's stress-response system is usually self-limiting. Once a perceived threat has passed, hormone levels return to normal. As adrenaline and cortisol levels drop, our heart rate and blood pressure return to baseline levels, and other systems resume their regular activities.

But when stressors are always present and we constantly feel under attack, that fight-or-flight reaction stays turned on.

The long-term activation of the stress-response system — and the subsequent overexposure to cortisol and other stress hormones — can disrupt almost all of our body's processes. This puts us at increased risk of numerous health problems, including:

- Anxiety
- Depression
- Digestive problems
- Headaches
- Heart disease
- Sleep problems
- Weight gain
- Memory and concentration impairment

That's why it's so important to learn healthy ways to cope with the stressors in your life. Reducing or coping with stress more effectively will naturally decrease your belly fat. Don't discount how constant stress is contributing to your waist circumference as much or more than menopause and take measures to address stress.

Managing your stress is a little beyond the scope of this book, but creating the awareness of it and how it's contributing to your belly fat is paramount.

Is it harder to lose weight for women after 40?

I'll be honest.

While it's possible to lose weight over 40, it's not the same as when you tried to lose weight in your 20's.

It takes consistent commitment.

As you can likely attest, in your 20's and 30's, if you had a weekend binge and the scale read a 5 pound weight gain, that weight would be gone by Tuesday…In your 40's, that weight may take a week to drop (if ever!).

The majority of women have had a metabolic slow down, so you need to build up your metabolisms again. The good news is that building metabolism is not only POSSIBLE; it's easier to do than you think it is.

And even better news is that building metabolism requires that you EAT more. Obviously you need to eat the right kinds of things, more on that and building metabolism will be discussed in a later chapter.

The fact is, because you've had a little bit of a metabolic slowdown, you do have to have more consistent effort where nutrition and exercise are concerned. I like to say that we need to live by the 80/20 rule. What I mean by this is that 80% of the time we're right on track with our nutrition and our workouts and 20% of the time we can goof off.

However, as we age, we may have to adopt an 85/15 rule or even a 90/10 rule, especially if we're really far off the mark and we've let our nutrition, workouts and positive lifestyle habits slide.

Once we get back on track and get to a healthy weight, we can typically return to the 80/20 rule where we'll have a little more 'wiggle room' with our healthy habits.

The good thing is that we don't have to workout for hours and hours everyday of the week. I've got some great ideas for you to improve your physique and your menopausal symptoms that don't take you all day.

We'll get into how exercise will help you lose your menopause belly in the next chapter. But first, take a look at how exercising my way has helped these women who are just like you:

First off, I wanted to thank you for accepting my application into your coaching program. Over the last three months, I've been mostly unemployed and dealing with the uncertainty and stress of looking for a job and questioning what I should do next. I'm super glad I had this program to focus on and look forward to during these last few months as it gave me an outlet of positive change and control over my life that I might not have experienced otherwise. I've also really enjoyed interacting with you and the other people on the Facebook group - posting our struggles and triumphs.

Even though I haven't lost over 10lbs or lost several inches, I know I have transformed in other ways.

1) I feel motivated and inspired to do or work towards challenging exercises

2) I encourage friends and family members to get active and workout with me (sometimes virtually)

3) I have developed the habit/addiction of working out at least 3 - 4 times per week and a desire to maintain functional mobility for the duration of my life

4) I have a hunger to try new activities that challenge me both physically and mentally

5) I've made big improvements in my pullups! I can now do 10 pullups in a row!

Again, thank you Shawna for your coaching and inspiration to be a better athlete and a better me. You've given me the desire and tools necessary to live a healthy and challenging lifestyle.

Kate F.

I enjoyed the coaching community most. I lost **11 lbs and 18.5 inches** in the first 6 weeks. I also discovered so many healthy eating alternatives that I never even thought possible.

Kristi C

Chapter 3 - How Does Exercise Help?

Those who think they have not time for bodily exercise will sooner or later have to find time for illness.

Edward Stanley

How does exercise help?

First of all we were designed to move.

We were designed to be active.

The body does not like to be sedentary. A sedentary lifestyle is the reason you're experiencing some of your frustrating menopausal symptoms.

In today's modern culture of 'done for you' and 'automation', there's less and less need for physical effort of any sort. This being the case, it's necessary that we seek out opportunity to move our bodies.

Exercise, yes, is one of the 'simple' steps to losing your menopause belly and getting your sexy back.

But do NOT worry!

You'll not be required to run a marathon or endure hours of painful sweaty workouts to get the results you desire. Quite the contrary.

It's important that you understand this correctly, in fact, many well meaning women do the WRONG kind of exercise and exacerbate their menopausal symptoms.

But the RIGHT kind of exercise will turn on your metabolic furnace and in doing so, will burn off the extra pounds you've so desperately been wanting to lose.

Take my client Nikki for example. She's a long time exerciser, very fit, but still couldn't banish that belly bulge, she and I had opportunity to even meet at an event:

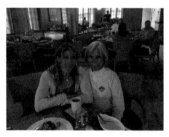 After starting Shawna's program, I steadily **lost 4.5 pounds** – but the exciting thing for me was that by staying with her program I've been able to keep the weight off!

What's cool about Shawna's workouts is that

although they typically start out easy, by the time they end, I'm sweating and feeling great. I have to add that I start each workout liking Shawna, I hate her in the middle, but by the end I'm saying, "Shawna, I love you!"

I had the privilege of working out in person with Shawna at a conference earlier this year, and I'm here to tell you that she is living proof that her stuff works.

You don't have to be a certain body type for her material, and through watching her great videos you can tell that this lady doesn't give up on anybody!

Shawna is not just for buff people, she'll take you from wherever you are and get you slimmer, more fit, and make you feel better about yourself.

Once you start with Shawna you'll want to keep on working with her!

Nicole Schweickert

Homemaker/Artist

The key to losing your menopause belly is doing the right kind of exercise to get your metabolism fired up. You've got to be exercising for the right amount of time, with the right types of exercises and this will create something called '**the afterburn effect**' or EPOC, exercise post oxygen consumption.

The 'afterburn effect' means that you'll be burning calories long after your exercise is done.

Don't worry - ANYONE can elicit an afterburn effect - this is not reserved for elite athletes.

When we experience that hot, sweaty and energized feeling after our workout even after we've showered, even in our car on the way to work, that is what's called the afterburn effect. This is our metabolism on 'steroids' - studies show that our body can be burning more calories with this elevated metabolism for up to 36 hours after we've worked out.

The good news is that we don't have to workout for long to be able to benefit from the afterburn effect. In fact, it's nearly impossible to workout with the intensity needed for EPOC if our workout is longer than 20 minutes.

Imagine an all out sprint - could you maintain this level of effort and intensity for an hour? Absolutely not. But it's this level of effort, for SHORT bursts for about 15 minutes that will rev up your metabolism and melt your menopause belly.

And this hot and sweaty feeling we experience during these workouts is NOT a hot flash!

Next, let's discuss what kind of exercise will bring on the afterburn effect, but more importantly, it's paramount to note what kind will NOT bring on that after burn effect.

Here are the first few guidelines.

We need to move every day of the week. This doesn't necessarily mean we need to exercise every single day, but overall, it's important to just become more active. Our bodies are meant to move and when we stop moving, it stops working well. It gets sore and stiff more easily, you'll lose range of motion and strength.

So simply MOVING more is the first step to losing your menopause belly. I call this type of moving 'active rest'. This means that we just make that effort to be active. Taking the stairs, parking further away, going for a walk, working in the garden, carrying groceries, scrubbing the floor - that sort of thing.

But, be cautioned!

A lot of people confuse activity with intensity so if you're just walking, or doing some of the above activities, it's not the intensity that you need to have that EPOC or after burn effect. Even if you're doing 'active rest' type activities seven days a week, it's better than sitting on the couch, but it will NOT get you the body of your dreams. This will NOT get rid of your belly fat.

These active rest days need to be paired with 'intense' exercise - more on that in a moment, but I need to clarify what 'intense' means.

Intense is a relative term. It can be personalized so that ANYONE can perform 'intense' exercise, no matter where you are in our fitness journey. Intensity is a measure of your **perceived rate of exertion** or RPE.

RPE is a psycho-physiological scale, meaning it calls on the mind and body to rate your perception of effort.

The RPE scale measures feelings of effort, strain, discomfort, and/or fatigue experienced during training. Our perception of physical exertion is a subjective assessment.

How is perceived exertion measured?

The level of perceived exertion is often measured with a 15 category scale that was developed by the Swedish psychologist Gunnar Borg. To simplify matters, I've chosen to do a scale of 1-10 based on the original Borg Scale.

See below:

1 - No exertion at all

2 - Extremely light exertion

3 - Very light exertion

4 - Light exertion

5

6 - Somewhat hard exertion

7

8 - Hard (heavy) exertion

9 - Extremely hard exertion

10 - Maximal exertion

To use this scale effectively, we must understand these things:

1) It should be clear that perceived exertion is a method to determine the intensity of effort, strain, and/or discomfort that's felt during exercise.

2) When rating your perception of exertion there's no right or wrong answer for the rating.

3) *Don't compare your performance with others* – So for example, if the beginner exerciser does a 5 push ups and this is their highest intensity, then they would give themselves a 9 or 10 on the RPE scale even though 5 push ups may only be a 4 on the RPE scale for the

advanced exerciser. The rating is very personal by taking into account YOUR personal fitness level.

Now, even though I mention that some kind of activity is required on every day of the week, it really depends on where you are in your fitness journey as to how much 'intense' exercise we should undertake.

For example, if you are currently fairly sedentary, it would not be wise for you to start intense exercise seven days a week. You could start with 1-2 days a week of 'intense' exercise and gradually work up to 3-4 days a week. A sedentary person might start with only 5-10 minutes of exercise and then increase it to 15-20 minutes of exercise three to four days a week.

Now that I've cleared up the duration and intensity question regarding exercise, I need to clarify what type of exercise you should NOT do.

What NOT to DO

Many women are fooled into thinking that steady state cardio is the answer to a flat belly. They couldn't be further from the truth when they say, "I need to do more cardio. I need to do at least 30 minutes of cardio to burn fat."

Studies show that 'steady state cardio' is the LEAST effective method of fat loss.

RESEARCH FROM W. JACKSON DAVIS AND COLLEAGUES AT THE UNIVERSITY OF CALIFORNIA AT SANTA CRUZ, AND THE UNIVERSITY OF CALIFORNIA AT BERKELEY, FOUND THAT INSERTING 'BURSTS' OF CARDIO IN BETWEEN 'BURSTS' OF RESISTANCE TRAINING YIELDED:

- 82% GREATER IMPROVEMENT IN MUSCLE GAINS

- 35% GREATER IMPROVEMENT IN LOWER BODY STRENGTH

- 52% GREATER IMPROVEMENT IN LOWER BODY ENDURANCE

- 143% GREATER IMPROVEMENT IN UPPER BODY FLEXIBILITY

- 28% GREATER IMPROVEMENT IN LOWER BODY FLEXIBILITY

- 991% GREATER LOSS IN FAT MASS

These are pretty incredible results: nearly ten-fold greater fat loss than just doing cardio alone. And when participants paired the bursts of cardio with bursts of resistance training, they also gained muscle at the SAME time which is very difficult to do.

Cardio is the most common 'go to' exercise for women. And while it's better than nothing I want to encourage you to change the type of cardio that you're doing. Instead of doing the low intensity variety for 30 minutes or more, try short bursts of only 30 seconds.

There are a few troubles associated with low intensity cardio:

- It's NOT effective for fat loss if this is your goal. Most women are interested in looking better in the mirror with all their exercise efforts. When this doesn't happen, many get frustrated and rightfully so!

- Low intensity exercise takes a long time. The most common reason for not exercising is time constraints, so finding an exercise plan that takes a very reasonable amount of time is going to be more successful from the start.

- Most low intensity exercise is lower body based (jogging, running, stationary biking, elliptical, treadmill, etc.). This presents a greater chance of lower body repetitive use injuries. It also does not address upper body strength or core development.

Now, if you love low intensity exercise, if it brings you joy, then absolutely do it.

However, just be warned that it will not likely get the transformational results that you're looking for to get rid of your menopause belly. You might lose weight doing 'traditional cardio', but you might just turn out looking like a skinnier version of your former fat self. I hate to say it like that but a lot of people tend to just get 'skinny fat' when they do just low intensity cardio. They don't look better naked, and that, at the end of the day, is probably what we all want to do is to look better naked.

I mentioned in the study above that short burst cardio is best paired with resistance training. Let me clarify what resistance training is and the benefits of it.

First and foremost, resistance training builds and maintains lean muscle tone. Muscle burns more calories even at rest. Muscle tone is what keeps our metabolism stoked and it puts the sexy in our jeans. Don't be concerned in the least about getting 'big and bulky' from resistance training. Women do NOT have the correct hormone profile to build slabs of muscle, especially women over 40.

Our body weight can be all we need to have an amazing resistance training workout. Don't think that you have to go buy a ton of equipment or that you have to go to the gym to be able to do resistance training. We can benefit with the added load of dumbbells, a kettlebell, a barbell, but effective workouts can just be done with our body weight as well.

Resistance training is actually what will give you the most bang for your workout buck. You'll get MORE results in LESS time, especially when we pair it with short bursts of cardio.

Women over 40 can and will build muscle with just our body weight.

'Old school' exercises like squats, planks, push ups, burpees - all done with simply your body weight will do wonders for your figure. All these moves are called 'compound' exercises because they use multiple muscles and burn a ton of calories all at one.

Let me be crystal clear about this: You do NOT have to do sit ups to tighten and tone your belly.

What you need to do is those previously mentioned compound exercises to raise your metabolic rate for your body to burn the fat off. Now there are some studies to show that local thermogenesis (or an increase in heat production) in a specific area will help to spot reduce, but for the most part, your body will burn fat off at it's own discretion, in the areas the body chooses and not necessarily where you choose. For that reason, getting hot and sweaty 'all over' is the best method for burning fat off your belly.

Let me explain what I mean when I say it's important to raise your metabolism to burn off fat…

Imagine going outside in the dead of winter in your warmest coat (I live in Canada, so this isn't a stretch for me).

What would be the most effective way to get your body warm enough to want to take off your jacket? Sit ups? Probably not.

It's more likely that squats, push ups and burpees, jumping jacks or running on the spot would bring on a sweat so that you'd want to take off your coat.

This is just like your metabolism.

I'm sad to see that many women throw money at their menopause belly by going out and buying a treadmill instead of getting on the floor and doing things like mountain climbers, push ups and burpees for free.

Or women are convinced that they need clunky machines to sit on to push and pull levers and weights to tone up. While this can be somewhat effective, most women wonder aimlessly around a gym floor from one machine to the next with no plan and they end up getting no results and then end up giving up.

Keep in mind that big box gyms don't necessarily want you to know that an exercise you can do at home for FREE is more effective than the sea of cardio machines they have to offer at their facility.

Don't get me wrong, it's 'possible' to get results on those machines if you have a professionally designed program, but the probability that you have all the correct elements for the most effective fat burning in place is slim. And even if you do have all the puzzle pieces all together correctly, you have the time commitment and expense of a gym membership that gets in the way of you getting your workout done.

I try to keep it super simple and inexpensive for ANY woman ANY where to have a solution to getting rid of and keeping off her menopause belly.

It's worked for me and my clients, it will work for you.

— — — — — — — — — — — —

IF YOU'D LIKE A SAMPLE OF THE TYPE OF WORKOUT I'M REFERRING TO, JUST TEXT WORKOUT TO 1-505-903-5242 AND I'LL EMAIL YOU A SAMPLE WORKOUT.

— — — — — — — — — — — —

Wouldn't it be fantastic for you to get results like these women? It's totally possible, just take a look at what women, just like you, have experienced:

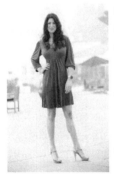

My name is Mari Carmen, I learned about Shawna K about three years ago and here's my story.

I am a certified Health Coach with a thriving business facing the bothersome symptoms of menopause for at least 12 months non-stop. It was bad, so bad that when I was able to tackle a good percentage of the symptoms by changing what I was eating I wrote a book to help other women going through the same ordeal.

However, something was missing.

I knew that science has proven that exercise is the real fountain of youth boosting your body's natural production of human growth hormone (HGH). But the way I was approaching exercise didn't feel like the fountain of youth at all.

On the contrary, I felt tired and run down, I was hungrier than ever and I felt that my body fat didn't want to go anywhere. The fat was there to stay and it was time for me to say goodbye to my beloved skinny jeans and pencil skirts. After all who wants a muffin top?!

It didn't matter how long my cardio sessions were or how many traditional sit-ups I did, my flabby tummy was not going away. So, I accepted my fate but kept myself open to find a solution.

And then came Shawna K!

I learned about somatopause and how specific body exercises could get to the root of my problem. Shawna taught me that addressing my HGH levels would help me look and feel younger with an added bonus; flattening that unwelcome menopause belly.

I used Shawna's scientifically engineered exercise sequences and literally melted my menopause belly.

Before working with Shawna I was working out way too many hours per week, had to use knee braces on both knees, I hated my long boring cardio sessions and my belly was hanging out of my pants.

After working with Shawna my knee problems disappeared; my workouts are now short, energizing and fun and my belly is toned and strong. I **lost 10 pounds** in less than six weeks and added muscle tone in places I didn't even know I had muscles (my belly included.)

I look and feel younger, but more importantly I have a system that has continued to pay dividends year after year.

I can't thank you enough my dear coach,

Love you Shawna!

Mari-Carmen Pizzaro

My legs and arms are stronger, I feel way better and my middle section definitely is smaller.

Natalie K *(lost 11 lbs and 13 inches)*

The workouts are a great start to my day and part of a my daily routine. I love feeling strong. I have energy. I have stretched myself. I have gained confidence and I no longer have that negative inner speak.

Michelle M *(lost 35 lbs)*

I looked forward to the workouts. The intensity in the 20 min is awesome! I gained endurance and strength my body is changing shape not just getting smaller. I gained muscle tone. I gained an appreciation for my body's abilities beyond my mind's limitations. I am really happy with the program which is very motivating and intentional.

Shannon H *(lost 6 lbs)*

I sleep better and have more energy. Thank you I truly enjoy myself and am happy with my **weight loss so far of 7 lbs**.

Tricia *(lost 7 lbs)*

I love the short but effective workouts. I feel better and more energetic, and I am now motivated to continue exercising and not lose the gains I have made. I learned that workouts don't need to take a long time and you don't need a lot of equipment. These workouts can be modified for any level of fitness.

Cheryl *(lost 2 lbs)*

I love the sense of accomplishment when I finish my workout. I always feel strong and capable! I have been better at setting and accomplishing goals unrelated to exercise, but related to my personal happiness. I believe it's all linked, the more I take care of myself and take steps towards the goal of being more fit and healthy, the more positive impact on all other aspects of my life. I recommend the program because I love the workouts.

JoDana *(lost 4 lbs)*

Next, in the next chapter, let's talk about the second step to rid you of your menopause belly.

Once you dial in the 'right' type of exercise, making modifications to what you're eating will multiply your results. Notice I did NOT say that you need to 'go on a diet'!

You'll find easy to implement, actionable steps so you know what to eat (and what not to eat) next.

Chapter 4 – Make Your Nutrition Count

Let food be thy medicine and medicine be thy food.

Hippocrates

Nutrition is a major key to your fat loss success and ultimately getting rid of your menopause belly. You can train all day long, but you must remember that your slim and toned belly is made in the kitchen with proper eating.

Making conscious and healthy nutritional choices is the second step to losing your menopause belly.

No wonder you may be confused about nutrition though because there is so much 'misinformation' out there. There's so much misleading advertising that it's easy to get befuddled. Don't get fooled into thinking that there's any kind of 'magic bullet' where weight loss is concerned.

There's NO magic bullet. Period.

Weight loss and maintenance success is just a series of smart decisions that you make one snack, one meal at a time. Not sexy, but the good news is that practically anyone with the will to consistently apply these tips will achieve success.

Keep in mind that this advice does NOT supersede any medical advice from your doctor. If you have a medical condition, then you might need to check in with your medical practitioner. As well, if you're not getting results it doesn't hurt to have a full physical (more on that in a later chapter).

My advice is NOT controversial in any way, shape or form, I am NOT prescribing a 'diet', I am simply suggesting healthy eating practices so it's probably unnecessary to check with your doctor prior to implementing my healthy eating practices. But feel free to check in with your doctor, getting a clean bill of health is always a good starting point.

I want to provide a few guidelines for eating. These are guidelines that I follow myself. As you may know, I'm in my fifties and these tips have served me well for half a century. You can be sure that I must be doing something right. I have loads of energy and I can trade clothes with my 20 something daughter. I wear the same size as I did in high school, I've had two children, I workout only about 40 minutes a day and I eat regular portions of normal food that I prepare myself. I do not survive on lettuce leaves and ice water. I'm no super star with a private chef.

What I'm saying is that I'm just a normal person and if I can do this, so can you. I suffer from the culinary affliction of being a long time kitchen klutz so the recipes I provide are simple and straightforward (and edible!).

I won't push hours of training or cardio on you, and I won't try to sell you expensive supplements, pills or magic potions.

However, I will try to educate you. I'd like to help you make smart nutritional and lifestyle decisions so you can enjoy better health, improved fitness, functional performance and even a flatter, more tight and toned belly that you'd be proud to show off in a bikini should you choose to.

Everyone should have a general understanding of the processes that are involved with nutrition and learn healthy eating to not only prevent disease, but to **promote good health**. Sadly, it's often only after we've had a scare from a doctor visit that we want to take care of our precious health – I'm all about education and disease prevention.

Let's get started…

Carbohydrate Confusion

There are many half-truths out there about carbohydrates: carbs are good, carbs are bad, avoid carbs, don't avoid carbs…on and on.

Diabetes is on the rise. As well, there are many people that are 'borderline' diabetic. Is your doctor telling you that you need to clean up your diet to prevent you from becoming a diabetic? Now is the time to discover what we can do to immediately lower your risk for diabetes while you drop unsightly belly fat.

Let me remind you a bit about carbohydrates so we can understand further how the body deals with them.

Carbs are our primary source of energy, as well:

- They are protein sparing. This means that they will be used for energy before other sources of energy (like muscle). This is important for those that are reducing calories in an effort to lose weight.

- Simple carbohydrates are short chain sugars.

- Complex carbohydrates are long chain sugars.

- All carbohydrates are sugar.

- All carbohydrates elicit an insulin response in order to lower blood sugar.

- Different carbohydrates digest at different rates.

- All carbohydrates are approximately 4 calories per gram.

Our body is a wonderful machine; if we ingest any kind of food, the body goes through a series of processes to break down this food. In particular, when we ingest carbohydrates in any form, the body releases insulin to counter the blood sugar rise that is a result of the carbohydrate meal.

Insulin is a powerful hormone that can be manipulated for optimum benefit. It enables the body to use the ingested carbohydrates in three ways:

- Carbs can be used as an immediate energy source

- Carbs can be stored as muscle glycogen

- Carbs can be stored as body fat.

Insulin is fat sparing; this means that if there is an abundance of insulin, the body will store more body fat. It makes sense then to avoid insulin spikes. **We don't want our body to be flooded with insulin because this makes it difficult to use body fat as an energy source.**

How is this done? How do we keep insulin levels low?

We will want to avoid the roller coaster of blood sugar spikes and valleys of low blood sugar. We have all experienced low blood sugar when we have the 'run over by a bus' feeling of low or no energy.

The 'go to' for most of us during low or no energy slumps is to grab a coffee or a sugary treat. The body will unconsciously crave caffeine and/or sugar as a pick me up.

In fact, smart advertisers play on this common occurrence. They try to entice us to eat a chocolate bar to help those mid-afternoon slumps. The result of this indulgence is:

1. A blood sugar spike and slightly more energy or alertness.
2. A surge of insulin because our body needs to deal with the added sugar in the blood stream.
3. A slump in energy, lethargy, sleepiness as the body shuttles the sugar into storage or fat cells.
4. An increase in cravings for either more sugar or caffeine as a 'pick-me-up' to get through to the day.

Does this sound familiar?

To avoid this, we will want to consume more complex carbohydrates, and avoid simple carbohydrates, or sugary foods.

One of the most effective ways to lower insulin response is to eat protein or healthy fat with any carbohydrates ingested.

Eating small meals five or six times a day is another effective tool to moderate the insulin release and control appetite. It's so much easier to resist tempting foods when we aren't hungry.

Try to eat every 2-3 hours, before you are ravenous. Then choose low glycemic carbohydrates, lean proteins and plenty of fruits and vegetables (more direction on this coming up).

One of my favorite sayings is *'Never Starving - Never Stuffed'*.

What I mean by this is that you'll want to eat before you get too hungry so that you don't eat the kitchen sink, and to stop eating before you're full. The reason for this is that it takes your brain about 20 minutes to register that your belly is full. If you stop eating before you're full, you'll be less likely to overeat.

A Word About Gluten

As you may be aware, there's a lot of talk about avoiding gluten for better health. Research shows that eating gluten can promote a variety of 'autoimmune' diseases including psoriasis and thyroid problems and may be the cause of a bloated belly, skin issues and other recurring health issues.

The best solution to finding out if gluten is an issue for you is to eliminate wheat and other sources of gluten including rice and corn from your diet for 14 days to see if you notice a change. You'd be surprised at how easily you can do this.

You can replace foods containing gluten with other complex carbohydrates such as sweet potatoes and legumes. The good news with this is that you'll rapidly drop belly fat and increase our energy as well. It's easier than you think. Don't be mistaken here, I'm not suggesting giving up 'carbs'. Just replace one carbohydrate source (those containing gluten) with another carb source (ones NOT containing gluten).

You'll want to avoid baked goods: pasta, cereals, crackers, and bread. There's hidden gluten in many other things like packaged foods and sauces.

Be aware of the 'gluten free' aisle in your grocery store. Packaged foods that are 'gluten free' aren't necessarily healthy. They may be laced with a ton of sugars and/or fats. The tendency is that when something is taken out of a food, it's replaced with something else to make it taste similarly – so if you want an 'Oreo cookie' for example, a gluten free one is likely not any more healthy than the regular one.

Now, if a full on reduction of gluten-laden foods is not for you, simply cutting back on them will make a tremendous difference to your waistline.

No matter if you're gluten sensitive, gluten intolerant or full on celiac, everyone can benefit from reducing gluten foods from your diet and increasing the number and color of veggies ingested.

For the most part, the majority of people KNOW what they should be eating; it's the consistent application of sound eating principles that throw them off.

Being proactive with your nutrition is often just a matter of paying more attention to it. A little education will go a long way to keep you lean, healthy and disease free.

More direction on WHAT foods to eat is coming up... keep reading!

Protein - The Unsung Hero of Fat Loss

My best weight loss tip involves a macronutrient that many people, especially women, get too little of:

PROTEIN: The unsung hero of weight loss...

Eating more protein doesn't mean that you'll be more muscular by osmosis. You're not going to put on slabs of muscle by eating more protein. (Women take note.) However, protein is important in the development and repair of muscles and equally important, protein is a big player in *curbing your appetite*.

Getting enough protein in the diet is no easy task. Protein isn't the 'fun' food.

For example, it's hard to pack protein with us when we're on the go.

Are you going to pull out a chicken breast or fillet of fish from your purse or gym bag? Not likely. Protein foods generally need some refrigeration and some prep time to make edible. Thus, there can be a bit of the challenge getting enough protein in during the day.

My suggestion is to add protein with every meal (actual snack and meal ideas to follow). As few as 10 grams of protein makes a world of difference and will help keep you satiated and craving free.

Protein helps stabilize blood sugar by slowing down the rate of breakdown of carbohydrates. Even the digestion of high glycemic carbs (simple sugars) can be moderated so that you don't get a spike and dip in blood sugar when you eat protein with any carb.

What does this mean?

Well, if you don't have a roller coaster of blood sugar, you won't get the highs and lows of energy and the cravings to eat the kitchen sink - or a bag of cookies, Mars bar, chips, whatever is most appealing and within arms reach…

This is one of the best weight loss tips out there: control your blood sugar to control your cravings.

Let's put some strategies in place to help…

First of all, you need to eat breakfast. If you want to be fat(ter), then skip breakfast. If you want to start to get lean, it starts with breakfast. It literally 'breaks the fast' of night time and eating actually stimulates your metabolism.

Here are a few ideas to help you sneak in more protein whether it's for breakfast, lunch or dinner or for a snack. Each has about 20 grams of protein (or approximately 1/5th of your daily protein needs):

- 1 cup Greek yogurt topped with 1/2 cup berries.

- 1 Slice Ezekiel (sprouted grain) bread topped with nut butter with 1 hard boiled egg.

- 1/2 cup steel cut oats topped with 1/2 cup berries and crushed walnuts and almonds and 1/2 cup Greek yogurt.

- 2 hard boiled eggs with 1 piece of Ezekiel toast.

- 1 full egg and 2 egg whites scrambled with salsa and topped with avocado slices.

- Smoothie with spinach, berries, almond milk and 1/2 scoop whey protein, 1/2 cup Greek yogurt

In case you were curious, here is the protein break down of each of these foods:

- 1 egg = 6 g protein

- 1 cup Greek yogurt = 24 g protein (I use plain Liberty brand, watch the carb content, many brands are just like ice cream with high fat and high carb counts and low protein, read labels)

- 1 slice sprouted grain Ezekiel bread = 5 g protein (I use Silver Hills Squirrelly bread)

- 1/2 scoop protein powder = 10 g protein (my favorite is BioTrust protein)

Protein at every meal and snack is imperative to your fat loss goals.

Here's a word on protein powder...

There are a ton of products on the market. Not every product will be top quality or agreeable with your digestion.

It's important to study the label and read the ingredient list of any supplement, particularly protein supplements. Ensure that there are no more than 5g carbs per serving. You typically do NOT want to drink your calories; you want to fill up with nutritionally dense foods. Supplement companies often use low quality carbohydrate fillers in protein supplements. Reading the label to see that the carbohydrate count is low on your protein supplement will ensure you're not ingesting empty calories.

Lose the Liquid Calories

First up, let's talk water.

Next to air, water is the element most necessary for survival. A normal adult body is composed of 60 to 70 percent water. We can go without food for almost two months, but without water we would only last a few days.

Most people have no idea how much water we should drink. In fact, many live in a dehydrated state, normally we need 6-8 cups a day.

Without water, we'd be poisoned to death by our own

waste products. When the kidneys remove uric acid and urea, these must be dissolved in water. If there isn't enough water, wastes are not removed as effectively and may build up as kidney stones.

Water is also vital for chemical reactions in digestion and metabolism. It carries nutrients and oxygen to the cells through the blood and helps to cool the body through perspiration. In addition, water also lubricates our joints.

Water gives us a feeling a satiation and provides the body energy to do all the 'behind the scenes' processes necessary for daily living.

Often times we confuse hunger with thirst. If you think you're hungry, it's always a good idea to grab a clear glass of water first to see if that quells your appetite. You'd be surprised at how this simple trick can save you hundreds of calories daily.

So how much water do you drink?

If you knew that it was key to your fat loss, maybe you'd increase your intake.

Scientists did a study on two groups of people...One group drank 2 cups of water before meals, while the other group were told to keep their drinking habits the same.

After 12 weeks of this study, the group that was taking the water before eating, lost 36% more weight than the less hydrated group. Their reasoning for this was due to an increase in satiety, that is, subjects had the feeling of being full and so ate less.

Do NOT drink your calories in the form of juices and soda pop. These are not only empty calories with no nutritional value, they do nothing to help satiety and can spike blood sugar so liquid calories like these will actually increase your cravings.

What About Alcohol?

Alcohol doesn't have much place in a fat loss plan. (Sorry for the bad news.)

Let's talk about what happens when alcohol passes your lips...

Alcohol is metabolized differently than other foods. It's not metabolized like carbohydrates, fat or protein. In fact, it's in a category all by itself.

Alcohol is a diuretic, meaning that it causes water loss and dehydration. Along with this water loss, you lose important minerals, such as magnesium, potassium, calcium and zinc. These minerals are vital to the maintenance of fluid balance, chemical reactions, and muscle contraction and relaxation.

Alcohol contains 7 calories per gram and offers NO nutritional value. It only adds empty calories to your diet.

Under normal conditions, our body gets energy from the calories in carbohydrates, fats and proteins that need to be slowly digested in the stomach—but not when alcohol is present.

When alcohol is consumed, it gets special privileges and needs no digestion. It simply bumps the cue.

Alcohol molecules diffuse through the stomach wall as soon as they arrive in the gut and they can reach the brain and liver in minutes. This reaction is slightly slowed when there is also food in your system, but as soon as the mixed contents enter the small intestine, the alcohol grabs first place and is absorbed quickly.

The alcohol then arrives at the liver for processing. The liver places all of its attention on the alcohol. So, any excess carbohydrates and/or dietary fats ingested are just changed into body fat, waiting to be carried away for permanent fat storage in the body.

Let me say that once more….

When you drink alcohol, your body will store any foods you've eaten more easily as body fat.

So you want to consider carefully that extra glass of wine

you have at night with some cheese and crackers, or that beer and burger or pizza you might have as a treat. The extra calories have very little chance of being burned off and more chance than ever at being stored as belly fat.

If you enjoy alcohol, simply cutting back on alcohol consumption to one to two glasses a week can have a big impact on fat loss.

Alcohol affects your body in other negative ways. Drinking might help induce sleep, but the sleep you get isn't very deep. Ultimately, as a result, you get less rest.

As we both know, sleep is an undervalued commodity by most people. If you're suffering from sleep issues due to menopause, the sleep interruptions that alcohol creates can be a huge issue.

Alcohol can also increase the amount of acid that your stomach produces, causing your stomach lining to become inflamed.

Alcohol lowers your inhibitions, which can be detrimental to your diet plans. You can more easily forget your goals one or two drinks in and really sabotage things.

Alcohol stimulates your appetite, so while you're getting calories from booze, it doesn't fill you up so you'll also want to chow down even more calories.

Here's the sad truth:

Booze: Lower inhibitions + increased appetite = Runaway train to weight gain

Those are my thoughts on alcohol, if you're serious about your fat loss, you'll put alcohol on the shelf until you've met your fat loss goals.

Keep in mind that fat loss is always a work in progress. In fact, even if you're not be trying to lose weight at all, limiting alcohol consumption will help you maintain a lean physique.

Small Steps

Don't plan on making sweeping nutritional changes on 'Monday'.

Too many people decide to go on a diet at the start of the week, and by Wednesday, they're ordering a pizza. Rather than taking on too much too soon, consider making one small change a week.

Most of us know what has to be done, we just need to do it. Consistently.

If you're too zealous at the start, you're setting yourself up for failure. I'll have more strategies in a later chapter on how to use your mindset to set yourself up for success every day to keep you motivated and moving in the right direction.

It takes 21 days to form a habit. It might be the wisest thing to make one nutritional change at a time. Work on a small change for 21 days, that will give you some time to get accustomed to that habit before you take on another one.

That way, you'll slowly morph your nutrition and lifestyle and you'll never really feel like you're on a diet. (I'll have more on goal setting and taking small steps in a later chapter.)

Finally, here are a few nutritional tips to keep in mind. You can pick and choose a few of these to implement slowly over time:

1. Eat Less than 30g of Sugar per day. The sugars you don't need to worry about which occur naturally in foods include: fresh fruit, frozen fruit, veggies. The BAD sugars: soda, cereal, candy, ketchup, syrup, juice, and many more. Check labels.

2. Eat Fat. Fat helps nutrient absorption, nerve transmission, maintaining cell membrane integrity etc. However, when consumed in excess amount, fats contribute to weight gain, heart disease and certain types of cancer. Fats are not created equal. Some fats promote our health positively while

others increase our risks of heart disease. The key is to replace bad fats with good fats in your diet.

3. Eat Good Fats: Olive oil, nuts, avocado, coconut, salmon and fish oil.

4. Avoid Bad Fats: Trans Fats. Trans fats are invented as scientists began to "hydrogenate" liquid oils so that they can withstand better in food production process and provide a better shelf life. As a result of hydrogenation, trans fatty acids are formed. Trans fatty acids are more commonly found in many commercially packaged foods, commercially fried food such as French Fries from some fast food chains, other packaged snacks such as microwaved popcorn as well as in vegetable shortening and hard stick margarine. They are on the decline, but it's wise to be aware of them and avoid at all costs. The body doesn't know how to process trans fats and so in an effort to protect itself, trans fats trigger an inflammatory reaction. Widespread inflammation is related to a variety of health issues and diseases.

5. Eat Protein. Protein is key to leanness. Increasing your protein intake will help protect your muscles from breakdown when your calories are down. Protein also stimulates glucagon secretion; this will help liberate stored energy. I don't mean that you have to sit down to a steak every time you

open your mouth, but there are plenty of ways to increase protein intake. Take a look at some of my favorite choices below:

- Greek yogurt (this is creamy, low fat, low carb goodness!)
- fish, fish, fish (coldwater fish!)
- egg whites, hard boiled eggs
- beans and legumes
- lean meats
- quinoa
- high quality, low carb protein powder

6. Snack tip. Include protein at every meal and snack. This not only helps with muscle repair and recovery, but it helps you stay full for longer because it slows gut emptying. You'll experience less energy crashes and less cravings. Eating actually stimulates your metabolism as well.

7. Drink Water. Dehydration is a killer. It makes you tired mentally and physically. Drinking water has a thermogenic effect so you will burn some extra calories while you hydrate.

8. Lose the liquid calories. Cut out sodas, diet sodas, and alcohol, fruit drinks. Get your calories from food that is more satisfying and nutritionally dense.

9. Out with the bad. Why tempt yourself and test your willpower? Clear all the chips, sugary drinks, ice cream, and other processed physique destroying goodies from your kitchen. If it's not there then you can't eat it.

10. Supplement with Fish Oil. There has been some evidence suggesting that fish oil can increase your basal metabolic rate and increase your insulin sensitivity which can help you stay lean and burn fat. Add that onto the boatload of data that shows fish oil decreases your risk of heart disease, eases joint pain, helps combat depression and alleviates PMS symptoms, and you have quite a powerful supplement.

11. No heavily restricted calories. It may seem logical to only eat a cup of salad a day; in fact anyone would lose weight doing so. But the body hates severe calorie restrictions and will lower metabolism by 30% or more on a heavily restricted diet. Your body basically goes into starvation mode and it will hold onto fat more than ever under starvation conditions.

12. 'Break the fast'. You need to 'break the fast' of your night with a breakfast that includes protein and complex carbs. The protein helps stabilize blood sugar, as does the complex carbs. You won't feel that energy crash at mid-morning and want to

reach for coffee or sugary snacks if you fuel up on the right foods.

13. Eat often. You'll actually raise your metabolism by eating. Your body will be more likely to give up those energy stores (junk in your trunk) when it knows food isn't in short supply. You should aim to eat every 2-3 hours so that you never get that 'I'll eat road-kill' feeling.

14. Plan ahead. Plan your meals and carry snacks. Who knows when you're going to be stuck in traffic or running late and need something to eat? If you have a few snacks with you, you won't be tempted to stop and fill up on junk food.

15. Switch to green tea. Green tea is full of antioxidants and lower levels of caffeine. BONUS: Studies show green tea helps your body burn more fat when coupled with eating right and exercising. (NOTE-Drink home brewed green tea - not bottled, "green tea", full of sugar or worse...artificial sweeteners)

16. Limit caffeine. If you're going to consume coffee or caffeine in general, it's best consumed at times when you're not consuming substantial carbohydrates.

17. Caffeine causes decreased insulin sensitivity and glucose tolerance. This means more insulin is released which means less fat burning can result,

and more fat is actually stored. These are three things you want to avoid if you're looking to shed those unwanted pounds.

18. My suggestion is to ditch caffeinated coffee on those days when you're eating a high carb breakfast. Instead, enjoy decaffeinated coffee with your carbs. Also avoid energy drinks and other caffeine boosters when eating carbs.

19. Know thyself. It's important to understand if you turn to food when you're stressed or want comfort. If this is the case, guard against this by finding other outlets to deal with stress.

20. Hormones? Sometimes the triggers for overeating can be linked to hormones. For example, the hormonal changes of PMS can make women crave sweet or salty foods. By understanding the triggers for cravings it's easier to curb them.

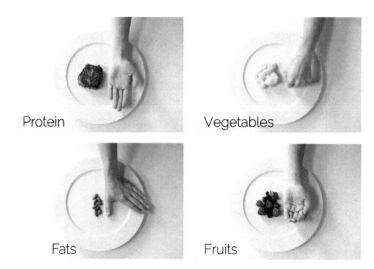

Protein   Vegetables

Fats   Fruits

22. What's on your plate? The main meal of the day should be a plate of food with a protein source such as meat or legumes on a quarter of the plate, a starch such as rice or quinoa on a quarter of the plate, and two servings of different-coloured vegetables on the other half of the plate.

23. Portion size. Watch your portion sizes. Over time, you can gain weight even by eating healthy foods if you take in too much.

24. For example, a serving size of carbohydrate is one fist. If a medium-size apple is bigger than a fist, it's two servings. Your hand is the perfect size to determine your perfect serving size. The smaller

the person, the smaller the fist, the smaller the portion and vice versa. Take a look at this diagram:

25. Step on the scale. Step on the scale regularly to keep weight in check before it has a chance to creep up. Regular weigh ins help you to discover how your body reacts to food. Pay attention to the foods eaten the day before a weigh in. Sometimes weight gain/loss can be attributed to water gain/loss, but by regularly weighing in you'll learn your body's rhythms.

26. Follow the 80/20 rule. Remember that you don't have to be perfect all the time. The key is moderation. If you practise healthy habits 80 percent of the time, then you can relax 20 percent of the time (but take it easy—one particularly unhealthy meal could undo all the hard work you've done for the week).

27. Write it down. Studies show that food journaling can be very effective in managing a healthy eating plan. If it goes in your mouth, write it down BEFORE you eat it. You're less likely to eat 'junk' when you have to quantify it.

28. The simple rule of promising yourself to write down anything you eat (before eating it), gives you time to pause to think. 'TOMA' or 'top of mind awareness' helps you to remind yourself of your goals and helps put a stop to mindless eating.

The smart phone app, My Fitness Pal is brilliant for this.

29. Be accountable. Find someone that you share your goals with and will possibly even review your food journal with you. It doesn't have to be a dietician or nutritionist, just someone that will hold you accountable to your nutritional goals. I'll have more on the opportunity to be accountable to ME coming up.

30. Go easy at night. Dinner should be the smallest meal of the day. You should also limit carbohydrate intake later in the day because carbohydrate tolerance is at its lowest point in the evening. This means that your body will store fat more readily later in the day.

31. It's a marathon and not a sprint. These changes should be implemented slowly over time. Healthy eating habits are geared for the long haul, not something that will stop as a diet does.

32. Grocery shopping: Make a list and stick to it – If you know what you need, you're less likely to shop for things you don't need. If an item isn't on your list, it may be because it doesn't fit with your plan.

33. Grocery shopping: Shop outside – The perimeter that is. All the best foods are on the perimeter of the

store, and the less nutritious and more processed foods are on the shelves.

34. Grocery shopping: Don't go hungry! – Everything looks yummy and tempting on an empty stomach. Avoid this by eating before you go shopping.

35. Mindful eating - Don't eat in front of the TV or in your car. Be mindful of when you feel satisfied. Stop eating before you're full, and start eating before you're famished. You want to be on this side of hunger, never starving and never stuffed.

These are just a few of the tips I use to help me and my clients lose and then maintain weight.

Implementing ALL these tips will be too much at first. Choose one tip at a time and slowly make changes.

Bottom line, if you want to see results, you need to DO SOMETHING.

Any change toward healthier eating is a positive one.

Even if the results don't show up right away – don't give up!

Tammy S (lost 12 lbs and 11 inches)

One last thing….HALT

This is a handy tip to keep in mind before ANYTHING goes in your mouth.

Ask yourself:

H- Am I really **hungry**?

A – Am I **angry**?

L – Am I **lonely**?

T – Am I **tired**?

If you're eating for any other reason than 'H' (hunger), it's time to re-evaluate.

Understanding and getting in touch with your emotions, appetite, and triggers will save you countless calories.

By adopting the 'HALT' method of analyzing hunger, you'll also have opportunity to make better life choices as you get in touch with yourself.

Lastly, the 10 minute rule...

If you don't adopt anything else, the 10 minute rule is an easy principle to apply where nutrition is concerned.

If you're ever tempted to have a second helping, indulge in a dessert, or put your hand in the cookie jar or cracker box, (insert temptation here…) set your timer for 10 minutes.

Do not indulge until your timer goes off.

During that window of 10 minutes, it's quite likely that you'll change your mind and resist the temptation. You'll have time to think about your goals, ask yourself if you're really hungry or if the temptation is really worth indulging in.

And you may discover that you really ARE hungry, in which case, go ahead and eat.

Remember: It's the SMALL steps that you take to improve your nutrition that will take you the furthest in your journey.

Speaking of 'small changes', I wanted to share a story of a rock star client, Diane. Over the course of a year, she lost over 50 pounds and it all started with ONE small change.

> Diane knew that she needed to make changes to her nutrition but she decided that she would do ONE thing and then build on it. This was a BRILLIANT approach because the changes she chose to make were doable, easy to remember and she never felt deprived.

Her very first change was that she stopped putting sugar in her coffee and tea. Did this help her magically lose 50 lbs? No. But it was a tiny step in the right direction. She was able to easily comply to this 'rule' she set out for herself.

The next change was that she swapped out her brand of yogurt. She read labels and found one with higher protein and less sugar. What this the magic bullet? No, this was not the magic bullet that helped her lose her weight, but this small change on top of no sugar in tea and coffee, and a number of other small doable changes that she implemented over time were what made her successful.

She also included metabolic resistance training - the kind that I talked about in the previous chapter. Short burst cardio paired with muscle strengthening resistance training changed her body so that she looks entirely different now.

She focused on the mirror and not the scale. She used her clothes to judge whether she was making progress, when the waistband on her pants was looser, she knew she was making progress.

The thing is, as mentioned in a previous chapter, the scale doesn't tell the whole story. Diane was losing fat and gaining a little muscle tone simultaneously, so the scale may have read the same number on some days. She did not get discouraged. No matter what, she knew that the proper nutrition and the right exercise that she was implementing was imperative for improved health, even if the mirror did not reflect the ideal image some days.

Diane is an excellent example that no matter what your age, you can improve your health and lose fat. Diane is in her late fifties. She is a rock star!

If Diane can do it, so can you.

Want a nutrition plan for you to get started with?

Realistically I don't want you to have to rely on a written out meal plan to live by day by day. Ultimately, we want to learn to make better nutritional choices so that eventually we don't need a meal plan or cheat sheet to follow at all. Ultimately we'll just KNOW what to eat and when to eat it.

But you need to start somewhere and I have just the thing.

You will establish better eating habits with this free Paleo meal plan and recipes I have for you.

JUST TEXT THE WORD PALEO TO 1-505-903-5242

FOLLOW THE PROMPTS SENT AND YOU'LL BE
EMAILED 'GO PALEO!'. THIS IS A RDA CREATED
'READ IT AND EAT IT' NUTRITION PLAN AND
RECIPE BOOK.

In the next chapter, you'll discover some common things
that might actually be the cause of your menopause
symptoms. There's more good news ahead because
you'll find that you can do a lot to take control and end
your suffering.

Chapter 5 – Sleep and Other Menopause Mysteries

Exhaustion makes wimps out of all of us.

James Loehr

Sleep Your Way Thin

Are you getting enough sleep? Have you ever thought that burning the midnight oil is actually making you fat? It's true. The fact is that if you're sleep deprived, you're also depriving your body of the opportunity to recover and provide the right environment to support your efforts to lose those extra pounds.

Oftentimes, lack of sleep will cause stress for the body. In times of stress, the body's reaction is to release 'cortisol'. This is the powerful hormone that increases body fat, especially that fat around the midsection that so many of you are trying to reduce.

In healthy, rested individuals, human growth hormone (HGH) is released in the body about every 45 minutes, but most HGH is released in the deepest levels of sleep. Growth hormone has an important effect on your metabolism. Efficient HGH production decreases body fat and increases lean muscle.

If you aren't getting the correct amount of sleep, your body never gets into the deepest levels of sleep and you produce less HGH. As we age, we naturally produce less HGH anyways, so it's important that we maximize HGH production to receive any benefits from it in terms of staying healthy.

Sleep is often seen as a luxury rather than a necessity for healthy living.

Many people are over scheduled and what seems to be undervalued and shrinking from the day-timer is valuable rest. Studies show that those that regularly get less sleep have an increased chance of obesity. Healthy sleeping habits are as important as proper eating and exercise.

Here are a few tips on developing and maintaining a good bedtime routine:

- Avoid caffeinated products later in the day.

- Avoid alcohol as a sleep aid.

- Avoid heavy exercise right before bed.

- Avoid <u>long</u> mid-day naps as this interrupts the 24 hour sleep cycle and can affect the quality of sleep you have at night.

- Develop a routine to help the mind and body slow down before retiring.

- Make your room as dark as possible as this will increase the secretion of melatonin which helps you to get into the deeper stages of sleep.

- Maintain a regular schedule as much as possible. Late nights and sleeping in on weekends can throw off your body clock.

- Exercise regularly and maintain sensible eating habits.

You may surprise yourself at how much better you feel with regular sleeping habits.

When better rested, there's also the added benefit of more energy to devote to all your other pursuits, including your fitness and weight loss goals. I'm convinced that some people don't know what they're missing or don't know how good it feels to be truly rested. It's a sad reflection on our 24/7 society that devoting 7-8 hours a night to the pillow is seen as wasteful - but that's a topic for another day.

Wait a minute! I know what you're thinking….

By now you may KNOW the benefits of sleep, you're just not getting any with your angry menopausal symptoms….

Here's the good news…

When you address other areas of your life, like your need for exercise and healthy nutrition, sleep will come more easily.

Will you sleep like a baby? Yes, sometimes. Other times, not so much. But you can increase the quality of your sleep an enormous amount by improving your lifestyle habits.

For those of you that suffer from sleep issues, the promise of improving sleep quality is another huge motivation to improve nutrition and add exercise to our day.

— — — — — — — — — — — —

IF YOU'D LIKE 30 WAYS TO IMPROVE SLEEP, I HAVE A HANDY CALENDAR WITH 30 MORE WAYS TO IMPROVE YOUR SLEEP QUALITY AND ENVIRONMENT.

JUST TEXT SLEEP TO 1-505-903-5242

— — — — — — — — — — — —

Insulin resistance

Many women are suffering needlessly because a lot of

menopausal symptoms are actually confused with insulin resistance.

What is insulin?

Insulin is a hormone produced specifically by the pancreas. Insulin helps the body to metabolize (process) carbohydrates, fats, and proteins from the diet. It's necessary to move sugar from the blood into other body tissues where it is needed for energy. Cells cannot utilize glucose without insulin.

It should be noted that it's not possible to use fat as an energy source when you have a surge of insulin in your blood. Since most of us are interested in losing belly fat, this is another reason why we need to keep insulin surges under control - you can do this by reducing your intake a simple carbohydrates (particularly in isolation without any other macronutrient like protein or fat) so to avoid blood sugar spikes.

If you are insulin-resistant these are some of the symptoms:

- brain fog
- high blood sugar
- intestinal bloating or just feeling bloated
- sleepiness

- **weight gain**
- **difficulty losing weight**
- visceral fat storage
- increased blood triglycerides
- increased blood pressure
- depression
- increased hunger

You can do a lot to improve your insulin sensitivity.

One of the easiest ways to improve it is to always eat a bit of protein with your carbohydrates to stabilize blood sugar. It's when you eat carbohydrates in isolation that blood sugar tends to skyrocket.

Eating fat and carbohydrate together will also stabilize blood sugar, but unless you burn off the ingested energy immediately, eating carbs and fats together is a recipe for gaining fat.

The carbohydrate increases insulin levels and the fat ingested is ready to be shuttled into storage if those calories are not burned as energy. You might want to re-think your evening snacks of cheese and crackers when you consider this fact.

The *primary treatment* for insulin resistance is exercise and improved nutrition. For the majority of us, we can control our insulin response simply by choosing foods wisely and adding exercise to our lifestyle.

Hypothyroidism

The number one reason for hormone imbalance in women over 40 is NOT menopause. It's actually hypothyroidism. Studies vary, but some studies suggest that up to 24% of women suffer from hypothyroidism after the age of 40.

Symptoms include:

- Fatigue
- Puffy face
- Joint and muscle pain
- Constipation
- Dry skin
- Dry thinning hair
- Depression
- **Weight gain**
- **Inability to lose weight**

Your first line of defense for hypothyroidism is to go to the doctor and have your hormones checked.

You'll want to measure blood levels of T3, T4, TSH and thyroid gland antibodies.

It's best if you're doing this yearly at your annual physical so that you have comparative numbers. This blood work will help to rule out the autoimmune disorder such as Hashimoto's disease.

Now there is a very wide range of 'normal' for the acceptable blood levels of these compounds. You may fall into the 'normal' range and still not be feeling 'normal'. Your symptoms might still suggest that you have hypothyroidism with normal blood work, so it's necessary that you have a good working relationship with your doctor so that you can work this through. Listen to your body and verbalize how you feel because even in the normal range you may not feel good and only YOU can determine what's 'normal' for you.

No matter if you are diagnosed with a thyroid disorder or if your symptoms are strictly the result of menopause, here are some additional steps to help you:

- Reduce stress
- Eliminate BPA exposure: Look for BPA free water bottles and avoid the use of plastic food containers in the microwave. In one study, women considered 'obese' had 47% higher levels of BPA than women of normal weight.
- Fluoride can be problematic. Avoid tap water that

contains fluoride and chlorine. Use a water filter and avoid fluoride in toothpaste.

- Some studies suggest that UV filters interfere with thyroid function so check your cosmetics and buy ones with natural ingredients as much as possible.

- Eat coconut oil to boost thyroid function.

- Eat more magnesium: coconuts, brazil nuts, pine nuts, hazelnuts, walnuts, almonds and cashews.

- Increase selenium (eat 3-4 brazil nuts a day).

- Increase zinc intake (eat 3-4 oysters a few times a week), selenium also helps process any mercury in the oysters.

- Include iodine in your diet: sea vegetables, cranberries, organic yogurt, organic navy beans, organic strawberries, raw organic cheese, organic potatoes.

- Avoid goitrogens that block iodine absorption, these are found in packaged foods, peanuts, soy, soybean oil.

- Eat whole foods with minimal processing and organic when possible.

Following a nutrient dense diet, exercising and getting proper rest will not only help with menopausal symptoms, but they will also help with symptoms of hypothyroidism.

It's extremely important that you are an advocate of your own health. Don't blindly accept that you 'should' be feeling tired or worn out because you're in your 40's, 50's or beyond. Your energy levels naturally decline to a certain extent, but it's more likely that environmental causes or lifestyle issues may be the author of declining energy or health issues.

You are a smart women, you just need to pay as much attention to your own health as you would a loved one.

Next up, the power of your mind can be used to propel you towards your flat belly goals. You are only as strong as you think you are and I'm here to say, you're stronger than you might think.

Chapter 6 – Mindset Magic

Once your mindset changes, everything on the outside changes along with it.

Steve Maraboli

You'll Never Be Ready

Now as you embark on this journey, you may feel unprepared and just not feel 'ready'.

But guess what?

You may 'never' be ready, but you must move ahead anyways.

Change of any sort is hard. Whether you are changing your nutrition, changing to add fitness to your life, changing jobs, moving to a new home, ANY kind of change is hard. But we'll benefit immeasurably and feel more alive when we challenge ourselves.

And in this case, we'll be healthier for it.

I want to hold your hand while you jump into this phase, and I want to show you a way to measure your success so that you can implement change and ALWAYS feel successful. Now, I know it may sound impossible, but it's the perspective you bring to the journey that can be a game changer. When you feel like you're winning, you're propelled forward and motivated to continue.

More on that in a bit.

To begin, part of the battle is to remember to trust yourself when changes and challenges come your way.

Looking back, if you ever had children, ask yourself, did you feel ready to have a baby? Did you feel prepared to bring that baby home? I remember when I brought my daughter home, I thought to myself, "Oh my gosh, they gave me a baby? Now what?"

Or do you remember buying your first house or your first car or getting your first major job...did you really feel ready and prepared to take on all that came with those things?

I remember when my now ex-husband became a

policeman. He put on his uniform for the very first time and we looked in the mirror and we just laughed, "Oh my gosh, you have a gun and you're going to be a policeman?" Even with all the training, he sure didn't feel prepared to walk into the role, but he did and he did very well at it.

You probably won't feel prepared for changes either. But you must just take the leap anyways.

A Little Shawna K History…

I've done lots of jumping into uncomfortable places over the years, so I feel like I'm well versed to discuss stepping out of my comfort zone. I'll give you a brief history of what that looked like for me in the hopes that it will provide a little perspective and possible motivation…

When my daughter was less than a year old, we moved to the country. I didn't really want to move to an acreage, but we moved anyways. I felt isolated and alone in a big house on a big property with grass that I spent hours cutting because it just wouldn't stop growing.

At the time, I was teaching school part time and I remember thinking, "*I want to work with women. I want to help them feel better about themselves. I want to make a difference in their life that will impact their health.*"

I loved teaching children at the time, but my passion was

changing such that I really wanted to help their mothers. I didn't know how I was going to make that dream happen. Slowly I just started training women in my spare time, just one-on-one, just for fun, because that's what I really enjoyed doing.

I never had a huge epiphany of what that would turn into.

A few years later, we moved into the city. I thought to myself, *'Training women is what I like doing. I'm not getting paid much (or at all). It doesn't matter. I'm just going to see where that leads me.'*

I had so many women asking for help with their fitness, so I took imperfect action.

I was teaching school and I had young kids and I had little time for one on one training so I started 'one on twelve' group training in my home studio gym.

I realized that this group training in my home studio wasn't an ideal situation, I mean I could only help 12 people at a time. Then in 2007 I opened a fitness boot camp to help 30+ people at a time. I realized that there were still so many women that couldn't get in front of me, so I went online in 2010 to help women around the globe.

I should point out that although I had a kinesiology and education degree and a ton of training experience, I had

NO idea about running any sort of business, offline or online, but I felt compelled with this passion to help women, so I just jumped in. I sought out people doing what I wanted to do. I surrounded myself with the right people. I hired a business coach. I just stepped every day into an area of uncomfortable-ness of not knowing what to do.

I wasn't ready, but I moved ahead anyways.

This may be exactly the same as where you are right now. Whether it's with your health, nutrition or fitness journey, or any other journey for that matter.

The steps to success are similar.

And I have by no means 'arrived'. I continue to do uncomfortable things daily. It's a process.

Stepping out of your comfort zone, surrounding yourself with supportive people, finding direction through a mentor or a coach who provides a road map and to whom you are accountable - all of these things will help you get to your goal - whatever the goal may be.

Let me focus on the difference between a support network and a mentor.

We need both.

Our support network motivates and encourages us, but our coach holds us accountable. While our support network can be a shoulder to lean on, the coach holds our feet to the fire to push and challenge us to press on.

Doors open when you take action.

For me, since I'm very introverted, it would be much easier to sit behind my laptop, but I know that I'd miss out on so many opportunities if I stay where it's 'safe'.

Every time I do a video, Facebook Live, interview, webinar, meet a new person, go to a live event...these are things that I struggle with. But I put on my big girl pants and just do them anyways. I can't do what I need to do without stepping into these scary places. And doing these things gets easier all the time because practice makes perfect.

I can recall going to one event in particular and I really just wanted to stay in my room because I didn't know a soul. My feet had other ideas though, they just started walking down to the conference room. My feet knew that if they went, the rest of me would have to follow. And it was fine; I did what I needed to do. The next time I'm in a similar situation, I know I'll be able to count on my feet to move me in the right direction.

I'm not special in any way, shape or form. If I can do scary things, then you can too.

Step Out of Your Comfort Zone

I understand that starting a journey to better health is a big scary step.

You've taken the first step, and that is to pick up this book and start to find the support you need. It's important that you prioritize yourself and your health for a change.

Women are the caregivers of the world but we often are the last people on the list to be cared for. Between making dinner, or caring for a child or a parent or driving someone somewhere, volunteering, working, cleaning the house, walking the dog or changing the cat litter... when on earth is there time?

There is always something to do; we often don't have time to think about our own needs much of the time. But the thing is, when we take care of 'us', our world improves because of that 'ripple effect' I mentioned in chapter one. When we're feeling better about ourselves in our own skin, when we're healthy, our family tends to be healthier. When we're on our game, our families and our loved ones, our coworkers, our friends, they all feel that energy and they benefit.

So it's 'okay' to take some time for self care. In fact, it's imperative.

Ask yourself, 'What do I need? How can I help myself?'

and be open to making some changes, even if it means taking a bit more time for yourself. Being selfish to care for your own health will ultimately benefit those around you in the long run.

Change Comes Fast

The famous motivational speaker, Tony Robbins says that change happens with one decision. He says that the *process of change* takes a long time, but the *moment of change* happens in an instant. If you want that change to stick, you have to surround yourself with people that will support you so you follow through with the change.

And that's where I come in.

Having a coach or a mentor provides the 'tough love' you need.

Remember, the difference between a friend and a coach is that a friend will just say, "Oh, poor you." The coach or mentor will say, "Okay, poor you. Now what? What are you going to do about it?".

Sometimes having that tough love is really important, but so is having that supportive friend. If you have no one in your immediate area that you can lean on, don't discount the power of an online community. An online network can be just as effective to provide the support you need to reach your goals.

You can't transform your body without transforming your mind at the same time. So far I've **lost 12 lbs and 9.5 inches**.

Heidi D.

Say It Out Loud

It's important that whatever your goal is, you need to tell it to someone. Saying it out loud makes it real. Write it down, post it on your fridge, keep it at the front of your mind. And keep saying it. This is where accountability comes in.

I find that women will do almost anything for someone else. We take care of our families, we do our jobs, we volunteer, we're there for our friends, but when it comes to self-care, when it comes to putting ourselves first, we struggle. We tend to think we're being selfish, so we're last on the list. But when someone is depending on us to 'show up', in this case, for proper nutrition or exercise, we're more likely to get it done.

So tell someone about your goals. It would be ideal if whomever you told is supportive and possibly shared your goals so that you could lift each other up, but even if they don't, the fact that you're putting your goals out to the universe, will make it more likely that you'll succeed.

How to Always Win

Now speaking of success, I have a method to always seeing a win in everything you do. This is something I learned from a mentor, Dan Sullivan.

We're always told to 'set goals' but the trouble with goal setting is that we tend to beat ourselves up when we don't reach 100% of our goal and the majority of us are *never* satisfied if and when we reach the goal we set. Let me explain why.

Let's use an example…

Mrs. Jones wants to lose 15 lbs of belly fat. She is successful at losing 12 lbs.

When she looks in the mirror, she is discouraged by her sagging skin around her belly. Instead of celebrating the fact that she lost 80% of the weight she intended to lose, her focus has changed to improving the saggy skin on her belly. She never experiences any happiness in the weight loss. Her goal shifted (to tightening up her sagging belly skin) so she feels unsuccessful.

This is what usually happens. We make progress, but in doing so, we see how much further we need to go, so we don't celebrate how far we've come.

Dan Sullivan calls this 'The Gap'.

As we move towards our goal or 'the ideal' it continues to change. Our goal, or 'the ideal' is like a moving target or the horizon. As we try to get closer, it continues to move away from us.

Let's look back at Mrs. Jones.

She could change her perspective slightly to experience a legitimate win.

This would help keep her motivation high and keep her moving forward. She could look backwards to celebrate her weight loss and then look ahead to set a new goal to tone up her saggy skin.

We need to avoid the gap.

We can do this by always measuring our success by *looking backwards*. The goal or ideal will always be in front of us or on the horizon. It will always be moving forward as we progress. And that's okay. We're all a work in progress, we never fully 'arrive' at anything because we are constantly evolving. But when we look at how far we've come and compare that with where we started, we can celebrate a win.

> I have been singing Shawna's praises to my coworkers, family and friends. I firmly believe that a person has to be mentally ready to make a change. Make a true lifestyle change, not just a program to

follow for just a few weeks. Stick with it... Realize that transforming your body takes time and hard work. So far I've **lost 13 lbs and over 6 inches**.

Lori O.

Set the 'Right' Kind of Goals

One reason you may not succeed at your goal is that you're setting goals where the focus is strictly on the *outcome* and you may have little or no control of that.

It's better to set '*process*' goals where by YOU are in the drivers seat. The actions YOU take will determine if you're successful.

Let's look at an example...

Maybe you have a goal to lose 20 lbs by a specific date. (This is an outcome goal.)

There are many moving parts to making this outcome happen, some of which might be beyond your control. For example, you may catch the flu so you can't exercise. Your fridge might break and your nutrition plan is interrupted. Your mother in law comes to visit and your whole schedule is messed up.

All these things could add up so that by that specific date, you may not achieve the 20 lb loss.

We all know that this is just 'life' and more often than not, things can get in the way.

However, if you set a 'process' goal, you can be in control of your actions, even when life throws you a curve ball.

For example, you could commit to exercise four times a week. You could plan on bringing your lunch to work instead of eating out. And you could decide to limit wine intake to one glass on the weekend.

You are in control of each of these things; you can decide whether or not you'll exercise, bring your lunch to work or not or indulge in weekday wine or not.

All these ACTIONS, over time could lead to the 20 lb weight loss.

You can see small wins along the way when you accomplish each of these actions.

Speaking of winning, let's talk about recognizing your progress.

Celebrate!

Celebrating small wins is important.

Break your larger goals into bite sized pieces and give yourself a high five along the way so as not to get discouraged when things don't happen all at once. Where fitness and fat loss are concerned, sometimes things are happening on the inside and may not be noticeable immediately.

Stay the course.

Program or diet hopping will do you no good. You need to commit 100% to a specific course of action for at least 21 days to see results. If you only give it half your effort, you'll only reap half the benefits or results and you'll never really know if the program or diet plan actually works.

Jumping in with both feet can be difficult. That's why you need to ensure you have support along the way. It's important that your plan is more of a lifestyle change versus something impossible or ridiculous to maintain, like the 'cabbage soup' or 'maple syrup, lemon juice and cayenne pepper' plan. These fad diets 'might' garner short term results, but they do NOTHING to transform the habits that caused the weight gain in the first place.

Set yourself up for success by making small changes over time instead of trying to implement an overly restrictive plan or doing too much at once. Remember Diane from chapter 3? She only changed ONE thing at first, (no sugar in her coffee and tea) and this led to a massive 50 lb weight loss over time.

Making slow and steady with small doable changes is the key to long term success.

Gratitude

I'd be remiss if I didn't mention one last thing in this chapter. It's the ONE thing that helps me to feel 'happy' day in and day out; even when things aren't going as well as I'd like.

Long ago a cancer survivor and friend told me that he only has 'good' and 'great' days. This helped me put things in perspective.

This concept reminded me to be thankful for all the blessings that I might otherwise take for granted. Any day that I'm on the earth is a good day. Obviously, some days are more challenging than others; some days are only 'good' while some days are truly 'great'. When I practice gratitude, everything seems to fall into place.

Here are two easy practices that you might consider.

Before I get up in the morning, before I let the challenges of the day bombard me, I spend five minutes thinking about the blessings in my life. It's only five minutes but it sets me up for a better day.

Another simple hack is to retire at night with gratitude.

I have a 'gratitude' partner (or you could do this on your own). Before going to sleep each night, I think of one thing I'm grateful for and I text it to my gratitude partner and she does the same (or you could simply journal it). My gratitude partner and I don't read the text at night but it's waiting for us when we get to our phones the next day. It's a nice reminder to start the day with gratitude.

Speaking of gratitude, take a look at some of the messages that I commonly get from women just like you:

I Love 'Doing Life' with Shawna and the Women In the Group

I first met Shawna online from Australia about 12 months ago when I purchased My Bikini Belly program. I had been training for a few years but was stuck on toning and losing those last kilos.

Her My Bikini Belly program got me back on track, the program was clear, the workouts great and meal plans easy to follow. I was then keen to keep going and step up the workouts so moved onto some of her other workouts which were also great. My measurements were at last moving again.

Shawna is a great mentor who answers our questions. She understands middle aged women and she is 'real' with us.

The bonus with Shawna and her coaching is you get this great group of like-minded women who also help, support and encourage each other all the way. It is so great to be honest with these women. Thank you so much Shawna.

Lisa Coulson (50 something)

A network and accountability was key for my journey that made **losing 10.5 lbs and 13 inches** possible for me.Thank you!

Jennifer G.

Normally it's nutrition and exercise that I let fall to the bottom of the totem pole. I feel elated writing this as just now it is sinking in deeply, more deeply than ever, that I need to *put me first!* Right where I need to be in a self-fulfilling and not a selfish way. Thank you!

Jacqueline Z. *(lost 13 lbs and 15 inches)*

I never thought in a million years that I would be getting up at 5:00 am 3-4 times per week to exercise before a full day's work. I love it, so it's easy, thank you so much.

Darlene B. *(lost 6lbs and 18 inches)*

I have a fantastic tool for you that will help you identify

and celebrate your wins. It will help with realistic goal setting. With it you'll discover the secret to sticking to your goals and finally getting the results you deserve. You can use this easy step by step guide the guarantee success at reaching any goal in only 10 minutes a week.

JUST TEXT GOAL TO 1-505-903-5242 AND I'LL EMAIL IT YOUR WAY.

In the area of mindset and gratitude, I'd also be remiss if I didn't mention a recommended read 'The Perfect Day Formula' by my friend and mentor, Craig Ballantyne.

His book has been a game changer for me.

You see, most people are stuck and I was too. Every day we seem to just go through the motions, following our usual routine without ever stopping and thinking why we do what we do, or what we'd rather be doing instead. Using Craig's book, I was able to be more mindful so I could own my day instead of having my day own me.

Craig offers doable advice rooted in ancient wisdom. It's an easy read and one that I refer to often. The book not only helped me get organized, more importantly, it helped me prioritize what I should actually be doing to live my perfect day. If owning your health and happiness is important to you, The Perfect Day Formula is an excellent companion book to this one.

Chapter 7 – Work with Me

A coach is someone who tells you what you don't want to hear, who shows you what you don't want to see, so you can be who you have always known you could be.

Tom Landry

Now, before I go any further, I need to warn you.

At any time during this entire process of working to change small habits to improve your health and ultimately lose your menopause belly, there will be what a good friend and mentor (Bedros Keuilian) calls 'the suck factor'. Let me explain...

I've given you all the tools you need. I've provided exercise, nutrition, mindset advice and more. I've shown you success story after success story. I want to pump you up, inspire and motivate you. I want your success, possibly even more than you do! And because of that, I need to remind you of this one thing…

And that is 'the suck factor'.

This is when everything you do feels like it goes wrong. It's when you feel like you're not only standing still but you're going backwards. It's when the scale goes up instead of down. It's when you get injured and can't workout. It's when your schedule goes crazy. It's when the flu hits.

Do you know what I mean about the suck factor?

It's called 'life'.

The suck factor is around the corner. It will be there no matter what. It will strike when you're not looking. It will attack just when you feel like you're on a roll.

So you need to prepare.

You need to line your ducks in a row to set yourself up for success. Give yourself every opportunity to succeed by following the guidelines in this book and by surrounding yourself with the right people. Like Fran did…

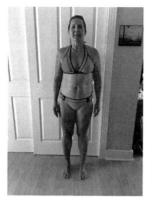

I've had the pleasure of working with Shawna and being apart of her coaching group since it's inception. It's a safe place where many like-minded women share their fitness & nutritional journey. I hasten to not say 'weight loss journey' because I look at it as a lifestyle change, it is permanent commitment to change your habits & weight loss is simply a by product of healthy habits.

Shawna has assisted me in making wiser nutritional choices & I have seen my fitness skyrocket. Her programs always challenge you to become more than you are, you never get stuck.

I sustained a serious injury (shattered my left arm) and even though I could not exercise, I continued to follow the nutrition plan and share my recovery journey with the group. It was a Godsend having these wonderful ladies to encourage me through this ordeal. Long story short, over 5 Weeks with no exercise, I pretty had minimal weight gain. This speaks volumes about how Shawna's nutritional protocol works.

I look to the future with hope & determination. I will continue to follow Shawna's program and participate in her coaching group with these wonderful ladies that I now call my friends.

Fran Michaels (50 something)

Studies show that if your counterparts are overweight, there's a greater likelihood that you will be overweight too. The opposite is also true. When you surround yourself with other like-minded people, you can support and uplift each other.

Listen, I know your situation.

You may have all the best of intentions and you may have been chasing that elusive pant size for a long time. You've may have tried to diet and exercise.

Nothing seems to work. *That's why you're reading this book.*

You may even have an exercise program that you've been following, but it doesn't seem to help you reach your goals. It's either your diet that's off or the exercise routine that's not quite right.

In any case, you're not successful… So many of my clients feel this way and they've told me:

If only I had you following me around, I could stay on track. I could reach my fitness and fat loss goals.

I listened and found a solution….

You have a busy life and don't have time to figure out what to eat or what workout to do. Decision fatigue sets in and you may end up not doing anything at all.

You need to have some direction from someone who lives in your shoes. It's difficult to take some 20-something trainer's advice. How on earth would he or she have a clue about your issues?

Well, we live parallel lives and I've created a program that will make it easy for you to follow.

I've been listening and reading your emails. I understand your struggles; in fact, I'm living many of them. And because I truly want to see you experience the lifelong results you deserve…I've created the **ultimate support system** for you because together we can do so much more than when we're on our own…

Imagine if you had:

- Direction with your nutrition and workouts

- Fresh follow along workouts monthly
- Social support and accountability
- Yummy recipes to follow each week
- Motivational emails and videos to your inbox
- 247 contact with me and a group of like-minded women

Imagine if I could hold your hand every step of the way to:

- Stop yo yo dieting, lose weight and keep it off for good.
- Abandon the fear of re-gaining weight and experience control for the first time.
- Understand the links to why you gained weight in the first place and what to do about it.
- Know why other attempts at fat loss have failed.
- Discover why you feel hungry all the time, have horrible cravings and can't make progress.
- Understand the neuroscience that causes self-sabotage to set yourself up for long term success.
- Understand what foods make you feel full and satisfied so that you are never starving.
- Reduce cravings and mood swings so you lose

weight long term->Stop binge eating for good and feel in control.

- Break free of the constant battle with food and weight gain and enjoy long term consistency.
- Feel fully supported with enjoyable, age appropriate, do at home exercise follow along videos.
- *FINALLY take charge of your future and health.*

Look, my time is pretty short these days with running multiple online and offline businesses.

In addition to coaching women like you, I consult with other businesses to help them reach women through improved health, nutrition and fitness too. You see, I have a mission to help 100,000 women get healthier and I can't do it alone. The way I see it, when I help other trainers improve the lives and health of women, the sooner I'll reach my goal of helping 100K women.

So I developed something to touch the lives of people like you and harness the power of a community to help.

You see, women are fortunate in that we tend to lean on and support each other - even total strangers. I've created a safe place that provides the direction you need and I've set the tone so that a beautiful community of women, just like you, has developed. Not only do people lean on each other, it's this community and accountability that has pushed them towards their goals.

Here's a sample of some progress from within the group:

Shawna Kaminski
Let's do a collective weight loss tally, can you chime in with how many pounds and inches you're down after phase 1 (21 days)?

This is NOT a competition to all you super competitive people out there!
(Lisa Bullock, Lisa Fulton). Some of you (Suzie Salmon) had other goals, like seeing visible abs and doing a pull up (Lisa Fulton) and these are just as important and legit.

Like · Comment · 13 hours ago near Calgary

👍 Stephanie Wright Pool, Laura Hampton and 2 others ✔ Seen by 22 like this.

> **Suzie Salmon** Good morning Shawna ! Can I have my coffee first? Lol
> · Unlike · 👍 2

> **CathyJo Fields** 6lbs. 7 5/8 inches
> · Unlike · 👍 1

> **Cris Lee** 6lbs 13 inches
> · Unlike · 👍 3

> **Katherine Dusik** 14 lbs./5 inches
> · Unlike · 👍 3

> **Laura Hampton** 4.4lbs, 9.7 inches
> · Unlike · 👍 3

> **Suzie Salmon** 6.4 lb and 2 3/4" (1/4" from each bicep, 1/2" from waist, 3/4" from abdomen, and 1" from hips).
> 11 hours ago · Unlike · 👍 8

> **Teresa Gillies** 6 pounds lost and 10.5 inches

Lisa Fulton 7 lbs and 4.7 inches. And contrary to what Shawna says I'm really not that competitive! It's just a Lisa thing. (right Lisa Bullock??)
10 hours ago · Unlike · 👍 8

 Karen Rogers 8lbs (7.92 to be exact). 10 inches. I'll own up to being competitive but I think we're all winners here.
9 hours ago · Unlike · 👍 8

 Kate Vidulich Just weighed in and 4.1lbs down - lost 3.3% body fat boom!
9 hours ago · Unlike · 👍 7

 J. Emily Clark 13 pounds down, 10 inches lost and never to be found 🙂
9 hours ago · Unlike · 👍 6

 Kristy Bidyk 9.5 pounds. I haven't measured yet so I will get that done soon. Sick in bed today.
8 hours ago · Unlike · 👍 5

 Lori Dillman 10.5 pounds down, and about 8"
8 hours ago · Unlike · 👍 3

 Bruce Hammonds 10 pounds, 10 inches
7 hours ago · Unlike · 👍 4

 Lisa Bullock 12 pounds, not sure about km or cm hee hee. AMAZING results from everyone!!!!!
7 hours ago · Unlike · 👍 4

 Vaughan Carder 6.6 pounds lost and put on muscle size (which is more my aim) lost 4.5cm from waist and about the same from hips

You'll not only get the community, there's so much more.

I have a number of ways that you can work with me.

I have a small group-coaching program, as well, I take on individual clients.

I take on a limited number of openings due to the personal nature of my coaching.

I'd LOVE to work with you if you're the right fit for my program. All clients are accepted by application only.

Here's a summary of what to look forward to in the group coaching:

- Direct access to me on our private Facebook group coaching page.

- Personal dashboard so you'll never wonder where to start or feel overwhelmed with too much information.

- Expert fitness programming – including NEW follow along videos monthly. You'll never be bored or wonder about your workouts again. No matter your fitness level, you'll have scaled exercises demonstrated in each video. Workouts are short, intense and you can do them anywhere.

- Nutrition plan that is tried, true and proven effective with 1000's of clients. This plan and recipes were created by a holistic nutritionist. You'll feel satiated and have a ton of variety with this mix and match meal plan. This plan will not only get you results, but it will also teach you liveable eating habits for the long haul.

- Never be bored with your eating options or what

to cook. Your dashboard will be fully loaded with 21+ recipes for breakfasts, lunches, dinners, snacks, side dishes, appetizers and desserts. As well, delicious NEW recipes will be added to the dashboard every few days.

- Detox program & recipes created by a holistic nutritionist - This program will be strategically released at just the right time to optimize your health and fat loss.

- Interviews with experts - Get up close and personal and get insider information from leading experts in fat loss, nutrition, exercise and more.

And here's what you WON'T GET:

- An overwhelming amount of material all at once that will confound and confuse you.
- Sales pitches to more workout programs.
- 'Fluff' that won't help you meet your goals.

I've done all the heavy lifting for you.

I'll be available to answer all your questions, motivate and keep you accountable.

All you need to do is tune into our secret Facebook community and head to your dashboard for everything you need.

Even if you're a beginner, returning from an exercise hiatus or recovering from an injury, I have you covered. You'll LOVE the new 'My Bikini Belly Beginner' program. This is an exclusive follow along series added as a BONUS to ensure that you're fully supported - whatever your fitness level. This bonus can't be found anywhere else.

If you're an action taker who wants to achieve and maintain flat and firm belly results, this is the group for you.

Or, maybe you want more of a one on one experience, where you work directly with me. In this case, I create your nutrition, exercise and accountability program based on exactly your personal needs, preferences and goals.

The beauty of the internet makes both programs accessible from any part of the world. I have clients getting results in my own neighbourhood and across the globe.

Keep reading and I'll share how you can apply to join me in the Shawna 247 coaching group or apply for one on one coaching.

Think about it…

Has what you've been doing worked before? If you know that your efforts have failed in the past, it's the definition of insanity to keep trying the same thing and expect different results.

My promise is that while my Shawna 247 Coaching Program isn't for everyone, for those that are accepted, I'll help you reach your fitness and fat loss goals.

Guaranteed.

If you follow the plan, do as directed and if you still don't get results, then I'll refund your money.

But I need a promise in return, and your promise is that you'll work the plan. And the plan will work.

I only accept SERIOUS candidates.

The reality is that my coaching programs will work for you because it has worked for me and I'm not special, I'm just like YOU. If I can be fit & lean in my 50's – so can you. I've spent YEARS developing this program. I've worked with hundreds and hundreds of women that have succeeded before you.

It's your turn now.

It's time to break old habits. You may be excited to make some changes now but often times, tomorrow will come and you'll get back into your routine. Without any extra support, your motivation will lag, your old habits will return and NOTHING WILL CHANGE.

The way I see it, you have two choices.

Choice #1:

- Invest in yourself
- Get the support/motivation/direction you need
- FINALLY get the body you've always wanted

Choice #2:

- Do nothing
- Wake up tomorrow & do the same things that aren't working for you today
- Continue to be FRUSTRATED and possibly gain more weight
- Continue to be unhappy and dissatisfied with your body
- Risk your health

Take a look at a few more success stories from those that have worked with me:

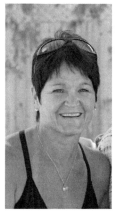

I am a personal trainer and even we need a mentor and I am so glad to consider Shawna one of mine. Her workouts are so engaging and give great results.

I love the camaraderie that comes with belonging to a group of like-minded people like her coaching group: Shawna 24/7. We give each other encouragement when it is needed. We hold each other accountable and we also inspire each other. It is like having an extended family.

Thank you for all you do for others you are such a giving and caring person.

Anne Schmidt

I liked the accountability of having to check in daily. The group members have been awesome, and I felt that I would be letting the rest of the group down, as well as myself if I fell off the wagon. As I started to lose inches and pounds, it made it a lot easier to stay on track.

Overall I have lost 10 inches and 7 pounds. *My clothes fit better, but most importantly I feel better.*

I have never been on a diet program, but I have learned about making sound eating habits, while benefiting from excellent, but fun exercise programs. The group becomes your extended family after a while. I wish the whole group continued success in the future months. Embrace life and enjoy each day to it's fullest potential.

Meryl O

Shawna K has made a HUGE difference for me over the last 90 days. This time frame included the tough food holidays of Halloween, Thanksgiving, Christmas and New Years.

I am 48 years old, and every year it gets harder and harder to bounce back from holiday weight gain. I was able to **lose 10 pounds and 12 inches** with a combination of effective nutrition counselling and workout modules that continually changed.

The initial 21 day nutrition plan or jump start was great for getting the program off and running, and I was able to put what I learned to good use over the holidays.

Probably the most effective part of the program for me was the individualized attention and support I received daily communicating with the Shawna and the group.

I was able to celebrate my successes with people who were going through the same process and had similar goals. And when I got down, skipped a workout or slipped up in my nutrition (movie popcorn, holiday candy, wine...), I had friends to encourage and support me (sometimes with some tough love!) to get back on the program.

Having to check in with the group EVERY DAY as far as motivation, workouts and nutrition also held me accountable.

It certainly is much easier to get your head out of a bowl of chips if you know you are going to have to confess to it later! Besides the obvious physical transformation, I gained an understanding of what works well for my own health and well-being.

I feel better mentally, have more energy, and possess a better attitude when I am eating clean, limiting sugar and processed foods and staying active.

Looking forward to the next 90 days with Shawna and the group!

Dana M.

If you'd like to experience similar success and if you're part of the 5% of action takers out there...Then go ahead and APPLY to see if you're a good fit for my Shawna 247 Coaching program or one on one coaching.

YOU CAN DO THAT BY GOING TO:
WWW.APPLY.SHAWNA247.COM

FILL IN THE APPLICATION AND I'LL GET BACK TO YOU SHORTLY TO SEE IF YOU'RE A GOOD FIT. I HAVE LIMITED SPACE BECAUSE I WANT TO PROVIDE PERSONAL ATTENTION TO THOSE IN THE GROUP.

And there you have it...the tools to help you exercise right, eat properly, set your mind and overcome other health issues.

Four steps.

Maybe they aren't entirely simple, but guess what? Living a life in an unhealthy body is far more difficult.

I'm looking forward to YOUR transformation and working with YOU.

All the best to you and your health,

Shawna K